WHAT TO EXPECT WHEN YOU ARE PREGNANT:

The First-Time Pregnancy Handbook,
The Gift of Being A Mother.
Discover Pregnancy and Birth as Well
As The Postpartum Journey.

HEIDI DAIS

TABLE OF CONTENTS

Introduction

When you are pregnant, you will see a lot of changes in your body, and some might affect your day-to-day life, but you will need to complete all the daily chores as life won't stop. What are some of the changes that you will feel when you are pregnant? What lifestyle changes do you need to make when you are pregnant? There are many things that you need to understand and learn. We will try to cover all these topics and prepare you for the pregnancy journey. You will be confused about whether you should drink or smoke, how often you need to visit the doctor.

You need to trust the doctor's judgment and make sure that you discuss all these issues with your doctor and follow these instructions to ensure a healthy pregnancy journey and safe delivery. You need to understand that your daily life will be changed and the sooner you adjust to your new diet, and overall health problems, the better it will be. Your new life will begin when you have a positive pregnancy test. This is when you think about the challenges that lie ahead and how you can manage your overall experience and pregnancy.

Stress is the first thing that you are going to notice when you are pregnant. The women who suffer from premenstrual syndrome understand how stress affects their minds when their bodies are going through different changes. The hormone shifts that happen during pregnancy are the most severe pain women has to face in their entire life. It is common to see pregnant women snap at the smallest of things and lose their temper. Women feel more fatigued during pregnancy, and this tiredness can increase the stress that they face. The women also face the strain of whether their baby will be healthy or not, and this stress affects their body and increase the mood swings.

You need to understand that mood swings are frequent when you are pregnant, and you should try to stay as relaxed as possible. Your friends and family should understand that you are not the only pregnant woman suffering from mood swings.

Many women think that stress affects pregnancy, but there are no reports where stress has tweaked the baby's growth. Stress is a very complicated concept, and every person has their way of dealing with stress. Stress level changes the hormones in the body. Doctors suggest that you need to learn to control the stress when you are pregnant as chronic stress can lead to increased blood pressure and preterm labor issues in women who are pregnant.

While being pregnant, you will see many emotional and physical changes in yourself. Some common changes that you will feel are muscle cramps, mood swings, and elevated stress. You may have felt these changes in the past, but when you are pregnant, you will fell these changes in high intensity. You will understand how these changes will affect your lifestyle and how you can manage them during pregnancy. Let your partner and your family read this to understand what your body and mind are going through.

CHAPTER 1:

Are You Pregnant?

Think you might be pregnant? You should take a pregnancy test up to 14 days after you ovulate or six days if you are using an early detection test. Any day before this time is not recommended, as it might result in a false negative. However, to ease your anxiety over the next two weeks, you can look out for possible signs of early pregnancy.

You might not get all of these symptoms as every woman is different and especially since the early signs are similar in likeness to the coming period. You can still refer to this list to check, but once you hit the 14-day mark after ovulation, take a pregnancy test just to confirm.

Period Pains:

Implantation bleeding occurs after conception is achieved wherein the fertilized egg attaches itself to the uterine walls, which may result in a bit of spotting and cramps similar to when you are about to have your period. This can happen anywhere from 6 to 12 days after ovulation and conception.

During early pregnancy, the walls of the uterus will thicken to prepare itself for the months to come, which will result in a thick white discharge from your vagina. This will be slight and should not cause any trouble unless the discharge is foul-smelling or itchy, then you will need to schedule an appointment with your doctor to rule out bacterial or yeast infection.

Breasts:

When conception is achieved, hormones change at a rapid pace. This will affect your breasts for the first few weeks of pregnancy, causing tenderness, soreness, swelling, tingles, or even itching. The nipples and the areola (circle surrounding the nipple) might also enlarge or darken.

These changes are due to your body being in the adjustment phase for the new hormone levels and should dissipate in a few weeks when you become more accustomed to the pregnancy hormones.

Fatigue:

When an increase in the hormone progesterone throughout pregnancy is first inhibited in the body, a woman might feel extra tired as soon as six days after conception.

Other signs of early pregnancy are lowered blood sugar level, lower blood pressure, and an increase in blood production, which could all contribute to fatigue.

Morning Sickness:

Morning, afternoon, and night sickness more like. Like most things in pregnancy, this again is all about the hormones. Hormones can slow down the digestion of food in your stomach, which might cause you to wretch and let it out again.

Cravings are also usual in pregnancy and with that comes the opposite, food and smells that you cannot stand. The slightest smell or even the sight of anything you don't like will be enough to nauseate you. Though not all women get morning sickness, if you have it, don't worry, it will ease at about the 14th week or as you enter your second trimester.

Frequent Urination:

Most women think that frequent urination is exclusively related to when a baby gets so big that there is hardly any space for your bladder. But it can be a sign of early pregnancy too. As your uterine walls thicken, your uterus also expands to make room for the baby. This will cause your bladder to become compressed and cause you to run to the bathroom at smaller intervals.

Urination Pain:

Any pain or burning experienced during urination when pregnant could mean that you might have a bladder or urinary tract infection. This is another common occurrence during pregnancy caused by the changes that the hormones have brought on, but typical as it may be, it is not normal and should not be taken lightly.

If you experience any pain during urination no matter how slight, see your doctor have a urine test done, catching this early will be better for you, the treatment process will be quicker, and chances of a healthy pregnancy are increased.

This might lead to more severe infection, further illness, and even premature labor and birth if left untreated.

Constipation:

As mentioned above, hormones could cause food in the stomach to not pass through at the pace they usually would. These same hormones (progesterone) will also cause the digested food to pass through the intestines at a slower rate, which will cause constipation.

You can ease this the natural way by eating more fiber-rich food or increasing your fluid intake. Ease up on the strenuous exercise for now, even if it is a way of relieving constipation, too, and check medication labels before taking anything.

Mood Swings:

Mood swings are frequent in the entirety for your pregnancy but will be most common during the first trimester, so don't worry if you go from being thrilled to be weepy. It's the hormones.

Headaches and Back Pain:

Back pain is another thing associated with the later stages of pregnancy, possibly because the bigger the baby gets, the more strain it causes on your back to walk. But back pain can be associated with early pregnancy and mild headaches that can happen as often as every day.

When taking pain relief, remember always to check the label and make sure your medication is alright for pregnant women. Better ask your doctor for a prescription or advice.

Dizziness and fainting:

Relating to the lowering of blood sugar and blood pressure paired with the dilating blood vessels to make room for the increased blood production, dizziness, and even fainting could be a sign of early pregnancy.

Knowing the signs of early pregnancy is useful in the sense that you know what to expect and the sense that you know to what extent these symptoms should be. Some signs may seem similar to the signs of early pregnancy but are untoward symptoms that can cause further discomfort and sickness, and that could put you in danger.

Vaginal Bleeding:

Spotting is alright and is a genuine sign of early pregnancy, but anything more than that should be a cause to consult your physician. Bleeding in early pregnancy could signify that the pregnancy is ectopic or that it may have resulted in a miscarriage.

Fever:

Any pregnant woman with a fever of 37.5 degrees Celsius or above may have an infection that may affect the baby as high temperatures, mainly in the first trimester, can cause congenital disabilities such as neural tube defects. This is part of what forms in the first trimester.

If you have a higher than usual temperature, see your doctor immediately for this to be addressed and treated as soon as possible before it might worsen.

Swelling:

Swelling in the extremities is common and normal in pregnancy, but what you should look out for is if this swelling occurs suddenly or is exclusive to one side of the body such as a leg, arm, fingers, or the face.

Swelling might be caused by blood clots, which are common in pregnant women, and you should see your doctor for treatment and further preventive measures to take. Alternatively, swelling might also mean pre-eclampsia, which increases blood pressure, causes proteinuria (protein in the urine) and causes seizures. In severe cases, pre-eclampsia has interfered with the provision of oxygen to the fetus via the placenta, resulting in newborns with low birth weights and other possible health problems.

Existing Medical Conditions:

Many medications should not be taken during pregnancy; however, if you have maintenance medication for a possible underlying and already existent medical condition, it doesn't mean that you should stop cold turkey and just leave it. See your doctor and ask for an alternative medication as conditions left untreated or not managed well could take a toll on your health, pregnancy, and even baby.

CHAPTER 2:

Your Pregnancy Profile

The doctor will share facts regarding pregnancy; the prenatal visits during pregnancy are frequent and essential. These checkups ensure the health of your baby. Bringing the father-to-be in the prenatal visits is vital as checking his family background and ethnic roots are also essential.

The doctors will have many things to discuss and need to make another checkup, and this is why; it may take more than an hour. The following visits will be shorter – such as 10-15 minutes. The frequency of prenatal visits depends upon your medical condition and complications. A medical officer recommends one visit every four weeks. The baby's heartbeat, urine, and body will be checked in this session.

Remember the date of the last period, and this will help in determining the due date. If you do not even remember the conceiving date, the doctor will do an ultrasound to know how far along you are.

Gynecological History

If you have not scheduled a preconception visit, the doctor will surely ask you about the gynecological history. He will probably ask about the earlier pregnancies and problems you might have faced. Understanding your gynecological history will let them decide how to handle your pregnancy. Knowing the complete medical history gives the doctor the confidence to handle your case.

Infertility Treatment

When you have used the infertility treatments to conceive, you should tell this to the doctor. Many complications need to be addressed when you conceive. There is a chance of multi-fetal pregnancies, and the doctors will prescribe the medicine according to your condition.

Medical Problems

Many medical conditions affect the pregnancy, and some do not; so, share all the information with the doctor. You should also tell the doctor about the allergies that you have. The doctor needs to understand your body condition so that you can give birth to a healthy child.

Family Medical History

The family restorative accounts of both you and the child's dad are significant for two reasons. To start with, your professional can distinguish pregnancy-related conditions that can repeat from age to age, such as having twins or uncommonly enormous infants. The other explanation is to recognize significant issues inside your family that your infant can acquire. Blood tests can screen for a portion of these issues, for example, cystic fibrosis. If there is a family ancestry of mental impediment or learning incapacities, examine the choice for Fragile X disorder screening with your primary care physician or hereditary advisor. Delicate X disorder is the most well-known acquired reason for mental impediment and results from a variation from the norm in the X chromosome. The pre-birth analysis is accessible for Fragile X disorder if your family ancestry recommends this plausibility.

Screening for Cystic Fibrosis

CF is additionally a passive condition, similar to Tay-Sachs. More than 1,250 distinctive hereditary changes have been related to CF. As of now, obstetricians and geneticists prescribe that CF screening be offered to every pregnant couple. Since the possibility of being a bearer is more noteworthy in the Ashkenazi Jewish and Caucasian populaces, screening (by a blood test) ought to be performed if, at any rate, one partner is Jewish or Caucasian. Screening for the 23 most basic transformations will get 57 to 97 percent of transporters of cystic fibrosis, contingent upon the ethnic foundation. (For instance, it distinguishes 97 percent of bearers among the Ashkenazi Jewish populace, 80 percent of transporters in the Northern European Caucasian populace, and 57 percent of transporters in the American Hispanic populace.) Speak to your primary care physician about CF screening during your first pre-birth visit.

The dangers of inheritable infections cover starting with one ethnic or geographic gathering then onto the next. Qualities get around among the different populaces at whatever point the guardians are from various ethnic gatherings. You can generally measure whether your parentage puts you at a raised danger of delivering qualities for specific ailments.

A few people don't know particularly about their ethnic foundation or family restorative history, maybe because they were received or haven't had a lot of contact with their organic families. If this circumstance is valid for your situation, don't get stressed. Remember that the odds that both you and your partner deliver quality for a specific issue are very low.

Thinking About the Physical Test

At your first pre-birth visit, your professional analyzes your head, neck, bosoms, heart, lungs, belly, and limits. She likewise plays out an interior test. During this test, your specialist assesses your uterus, cervix, and ovaries, and performs, if due, a PAP test (cervix malignancy and pre-disease screening). If you believe you likewise ought to be tried for the probability of explicitly transmitted maladies, educate your doctor because the PAP test doesn't screen for every one of them.

After the test, you and your expert will examine the general arrangement for your pregnancy and discuss any potential issues. Likewise, you can examine what drugs you can take while you're pregnant when you should call for help, and what type of tests you are to experience all through your pregnancy.

Looking at The Standard Tests

Prepare yourself: You're presumably going to be acquainted with a needle and need to pee in a cup during your first pre-birth visit. Here's a glance at the standard strategies, including blood and pee tests.

Prepare for the prick: Blood Tests

On your first pre-birth visit, your expert will draw your blood for a lot of standard tests to check your general well-being to ensure you are safe from specific diseases. The accompanying tests are standard:

- A standard test for blood classification, Rh factor, and immune response status. The blood classification alludes to whether your blood is type A, B, AB, or O and whether you're Rh-positive or Rh-negative. The neutralizer test is intended to advise whether exceptional blood-bunch antibodies to specific antigens (like the Rh antigen) are available.

- Complete blood tally (CBC). This test checks for frailty, which alludes to a low blood tally.

- VDRL or RPR. These tests check for syphilis, an explicitly transmitted infection. They produce a positive outcome if the patient has different conditions, such as lupus or the antiphospholipid neutralizer disorder. Nonetheless, these sorts of false-positive outcomes are generally feebly positive. These tests are vague, to affirm the conclusion of syphilis, another, increasingly explicit blood test ought to be performed. Since, fundamentally, syphilis is treated, ensure you get a check. Indeed, most states require it. Tragically, the rate of syphilis is on the ascent in the United States.

- Hepatitis B. This test checks for proof of hepatitis infections. These infections come in a few distinct sorts, and the hepatitis B infection is one that can be available without creating genuine indications. A few ladies are analyzed distinctly during a blood test.

- Rubella. Your professional additionally checks for insusceptibility to rubella (likewise called German measles). Most ladies have been inoculated against rubella or, because they have had the ailment previously, their blood delivers antibodies, which is why the danger of contracting German measles during pregnancy is so uncommon. Most specialists test to see that the mother is invulnerable to rubella during the absolute first pre-birth visit. An expert additionally encourages these ladies to get inoculated against rubella not long after they deliver, so they aren't powerless in resulting pregnancies.

- HIV. Since medicine is accessible to diminish the danger of transmission to the child, just as to slow sickness movement in the mother, monitoring your HIV status is significant. A specialist can generally play out this test simultaneously as the other pre-birth blood tests.

Ultrasound

Ultrasound utilizes sound waves to make an image of the uterus and the infant inside it. Ultrasound assessments don't include radiation, and the technique is safe for both you and your infant. Your specialist may propose that you experience a first-trimester ultrasound test. Regularly, this ultrasound is performed transvaginal, which implies that an exceptional ultrasound test is embedded into the vagina. The favorable position to this method is that the test, or transducer, is nearer to the baby, so a much clearer view is achieved with a standard transabdominal ultrasound assessment. A few ladies stress that a transvaginal test embedded into the vagina could hurt the child.

The precision of your due date:

Finding the time of the last menstrual period and a simple ultrasound test will help doctors find the right due date. The ultrasound test will show the baby's size, and the doctor may change the due date according to the reports. An ultrasound in the first trimester is more precise than a later ultrasound in affirming or setting up your due date.

Fetal reasonability:

The probability of miscarriage drops to less than 3 percent when the ultrasound test is conducted to check the child's heartbeat. Preceding five weeks, the baby itself may not be unmistakable; instead, the ultrasound may show just the gestational sac.

Fetal anomalies:

Although a total ultrasound assessment to distinguish basic variations from the norm in the baby ordinarily isn't performed until around 20 weeks, and a few issues may as of now be unmistakable by 11 to 12 weeks. A significant part of the mind, spine, appendages, stomach area and urinary tract structures might be seen with transvaginal ultrasound. Moreover, the nearness of a thickening behind the neck of the embryo (known as expanded nuchal translucency) may show an additional hazard for certain hereditary or chromosomal conditions.

Fetal number:

An ultrasound shows whether you're delivering more than one baby. Furthermore, the presence of the film isolating the children, just as the placental areas, indicates whether the children share one placenta or have separate placentas.

The state of your ovaries:

An ultrasound can uncover irregularities or growths in your ovaries. In some cases, an ultrasound shows a little sore, called a corpus luteal pimple. This is a blister that structures at the site where the egg was discharged. Through the span of three or four months, it continuously leaves. Two different kinds of blisters called dermoid growths and straightforward sores, are inconsequential to the pregnancy and might be found during an ultrasound test. Regardless of whether the expulsion of these sorts of growths is essential and when they ought to be evacuated, it relies upon the size of the blister and any side effects.

The nearness of fibroid tumors:

Also called fibroids, these are generous abundances of the muscle of the uterus.

Location of the pregnancy:

Occasionally, the pregnancy might be situated outside the uterus, an ectopic pregnancy.

CHAPTER 3:

Your Pregnancy Lifestyle

The health of your baby is tightly connected with your health. You have to make sure that you take care of your body because Junior will be counting on you to do this, and you have to be very careful with every move you make from multiple points of view. Here are some tips on maintaining you and the little one inside you healthy and strong so that you can have a normal delivery and a healthy and happy baby.

Your Condition Before Getting Pregnant

It is obvious that mothers who are healthy and fit before they get pregnant have more chances of delivering a healthy baby and, if you have decided that you want to have a baby, then make sure that you adjust yourself to this wish. That means that you should start embracing healthy habits as soon as possible because they can change everything for you and the baby.

Eat healthy, exercise, and keep yourself healthy in general. If you smoke, quit it. Don't drink excessive amounts of alcohol (and don't drink any of it during the pregnancy). Don't make excesses of any kind. Keep yourself balanced, healthy, and confident, and by the time you get pregnant, you will have less to work on when it comes to adjusting to the needs of your baby.

Cat Litter and Toxins

There are some pregnancy-related myths out there, but the one that says that pregnant women shouldn't change cat litter is not a myth. Stay away from the cat's litter as much as possible because there is the risk of toxoplasmosis, an infestation caused by a parasite. While adults who get infected with it will think they have flu, this kind of medical condition can be hazardous in the case of children and pregnant women, since it can cause miscarriage.

As for general toxins, keep yourself away from them at all times. They are not normally good for your body, but since you will be carrying another person in you and since this little person is relying on you to keep him/her healthy, you should make sure that you don't stay near toxins (and this may include hair dyes and hair perm solutions as well).

Also, make sure that if you are decorating the nursery room, you will not be hanging out near paint and wallpaper because the fumes associated with these will most likely not be healthy for you as a pregnant woman.

Listen to Your Body

If you need to sleep, then go lie yourself down. Normally, pregnant women feel very tired, especially during the first three months of pregnancy, and if you feel like napping in the morning, afternoon, and then sleeping all night, then listen to your body. There will be a time when your belly will not allow you to sleep as comfortably as you would want to, and when that time comes, you will look back and regret not having listened to your instinct.

Water!

Drink at least eight glasses of water every single day. Keep yourself hydrated now more than ever because your body needs it. Dehydration can put you to danger, and it can endanger Junior as well. You are allowed to drink other liquids as well, but you may want to keep soda and coffee within normal limits because they contain caffeine and contain too much sugar (both of which can damage your health and, consequently, your baby).

Take Classes

From prenatal yoga to childbirth classes, there is something for every stage of pregnancy you will be at. Pregnancy exercises, early pregnancy classes, yoga, childbirth classes, breastfeeding classes – all these things are very good to attend because they will prepare you for what is to come. They are the right way of coming in contact with a lot of people who may help you with information, with advice on where to find a good hospital and other such matters.

Stretch, Tilt and Keep Good Posture

You will be carrying a lot of weight in your belly, and your entire body may start bending forward. To make sure that you won't be extremely bothered by back pain later in the pregnancy, make sure to stretch your arms and back, tilt your cervical bone, and keep a generally good posture for as much as you can. Small changes such as these can make the difference eventually.

Prepare Yourself Psychologically

Bringing a little person into the world will be easy, and truth be told, the nine months ahead of you are just the start. You are about to change your life forever, and nothing will ever be the same because you will have to bear the responsibility of a little human who needs you for care, education, health, and so on. Make sure to prepare yourself psychologically. At times, you will feel downright terrified of what is to come. Other times you will feel excited. But no matter what happens, you will still love being a new mom, and you will want to cherish every minute.

Talk to Your Baby, Listen to Him, Read about Other Birth Stories

You must keep yourself positive and send the same energy towards your baby bump as well. Believe it or not, while the baby may not fully understand you, he/she will get acquainted with your voice, and this is where the unbreakable connection begins.

Also, it does help if you read the stories other mommies out there go through, and it helps if you have a more experienced mommy to talk to because many of the fears and anxieties can be alleviated this way.

CHAPTER 4:

Nine Months of Eating Well

Nutrition is the prime consideration during pregnancy. Everything practically depends on this. If you eat the right things in the right amounts, you are giving your baby the best chance to grow and develop normally. Not only that, eating the right things will help you to have a happy and healthy pregnancy. It will improve your stamina, your energy, and strength. It will also lessen some of the common discomforts of pregnancy, such as constipation and heartburn.

Calorie Intake

Additional calorie intake is only at 200-300 daily, not more than 500 calories. So, eating for two does not mean doubling your daily meals. You do not have to eat two servings of everything just to provide for you and your baby. What you have to do is to get the right stuff in the right amounts. Choose nutrient-dense foods like low-fat dairy products, vegetables, lean meats, fruits, and whole-grain products.

Balanced Meals

Aim to eat a well-balanced meal. It should include all the food groups in the right amounts. Make sure you get the essential nutrients your body and your baby need, such as proteins, carbohydrates, fats, minerals, and vitamins. These are all crucial for proper, normal growth and development. These are essential for the normal development of the baby's organs.

For you, these nutrients are essential to give you the energy you need during pregnancy, delivery, and the first few weeks after. Pregnancy and childbirth can easily sap your energy. You need to focus on your nutrient intake so you will still have the necessary strength and stamina for your usual daily tasks.

Getting the proper nutrients will also help to protect you from infections and diseases. Pregnancy is not the time to get sick. Even the common simple colds and flu virus can have severe effects on your baby.

You will need to eat well-balanced meals to improve your body's ability to repair injuries. During pregnancy, most of the body's stores will be used by the baby as he grows and develops. Only a small amount will be left for you to use for your growth and repair. So, you must take more to have more than enough for your own needs. For example, some pregnant women may notice that small wounds like paper cuts take longer to heal.

Also, a lot of pregnant women tend to have weaker bones. The most notable problems faced by pregnant women is with teeth. They have bleeding gums. They also feel as if their teeth are becoming loose or cavities begin to form. This indicates the body's store of calcium and other minerals are being tapped into and given to the baby. Eat the right foods in the right amounts to replenish your body's supply.

Components of a well-balanced meal

Experts on pregnancy nutrition have spent years of study to determine the right nutrition during this particular time of a woman's life. A balanced diet that supports the needs of the mother-to-be and the baby should include around 80-100 g of protein, water and salt, and enough calories from various food groups.

- 2 to 3 servings fish, meat, legumes or nuts, and tofu

- 1 serving of yellow vegetables

- 2 servings of green vegetables

- 2 to 3 servings of dairy such as milk, cheese, yogurt, eggs

- 3 servings of whole-grain cereals, whole-grain bread or other foods containing high-complex carbohydrates

- 3 servings of fruits

- 6 to 8 glasses of water clean, filtered

- Salt to taste

This list may seem like a lot but is actually enough to supply the needed nutrients for both you and your baby.

Good sources for the needed nutrients include the following:

Proteins:

- Beef

- Poultry

- Turkey

- Fish

- Nuts

- Tofu

- Legumes

- Eggs

- Soy cheese

Whole Grains

- Buckwheat groats (kasha)

- Quinoa

- Wild rice

- Brown rice

- Wheat germ

- Wheat gluten

- Whole wheat pasta

- Whole grain cereals

- Whole oats

Fruits

- Kiwi fruit

- Bananas

- Oranges

- Apples
- Pears
- Nectarines
- Plums
- Pears
- Cantaloupe
- Grapefruits
- Mango
- Peaches

Green vegetables

- Broccoli
- Dark green lettuce
- Lambs lettuce
- Asparagus
- Spinach
- Green beans
- Arugula
- Swiss chard

- Zucchini

- Kale

Dairy

- Cottage cheese

- Hard cheese

- Yogurt

- Milk

- Eggs

Proteins

According to the WHO (World Health Organization), pregnant women should eat at least 75 grams of proteins per day. Studies have shown that at this minimum amount, a pregnant woman can already decrease the risk for diseases of pregnancy like pre-eclampsia or metabolic toxemia that develops during late pregnancy (in susceptible people).

Proteins have numerous functions in the body. However, getting the right amount every day is not the sole marker for a nutritious and well-balanced diet. It has to come from healthy sources. Choose lean meats from organically raised animals, such as free-range chicken and cattle. Remember, anything in the food you eat can affect your baby. Stay away from meats that come from animals that have been treated with loads of antibiotics. The antibiotics leave residue on the meats and will stay there until you eat them. These residues will cause problems in your body and may affect the baby as well. Animals that have not been raised organically may also have been treated with artificial hormones. This is a practice among some livestock growers to improve the yield of each meat producer. But these artificial hormones prove to be unhealthy for humans, most especially to pregnant women and their babies. These can seriously interfere with the baby's growth and development. Other inexpensive natural sources of proteins include:

- Eggs

- Milk

- Dairy products like cheese

- Beans

- Soybeans

- Soy products

- Nuts

CHAPTER 5:

The First Month

Weeks 1 and 2

During weeks 1 and 2, you might not consider yourself pregnant. The conception likely hasn't even happened yet during this point. Your body will go through the usual menstrual cycle during the first week, getting rid of the unfertilized last month and preparing itself for the next egg.

During this, your body will prepare the egg to be released into the fallopian tube. All of this is coordinated by the hormones that regulate your body. Eggs are contained in follicles. The first step is the follicle stimulating hormone (FSH). When the follicles mature, they produce estrogen and progesterone. These two hormones signal to your body to begin repairing the uterus and thickening the walls. The estrogen will eventually trigger the luteinizing hormone (LH). LH will cause the most mature egg to leave the follicle. This usually occurs 24-36 hours after LH levels spike in the body. This spike occurs roughly two weeks, sometimes slightly less, into the cycle. This is ovulation. Your body is then prepared for the sperm to fertilize the egg.

While the ovum, the egg, heads down your fallopian tube, your body will use estrogen to start the process of getting your uterine wall to thicken. A blood-rich lining will fill the wall of the uterus. At this point in the cycle, some women feel one-sided pain. There's also breast soreness, heavy boobs, as well as mild cramp and PMS.

During this period in the cycle, a woman may be particularly sensitive to smells. The progesterone hormone will help the fertilized egg take hold of the uterine wall if conception happens. During the first weeks, you may be thinking about the dietary and health concerns you should be focusing on even if you're not pregnant.

Week 3

In the third week, a single sperm cell conjoins with the ovum that has been expelled from the ovaries during ovulation, and this results in conception. The fertilization of the egg in the fallopian tube can occur anywhere from 45 minutes to seven days after sexual activity. The average amount of time it takes for a sperm to find an egg is around twelve hours, but the quickest of the sperm can do so within 45 minutes. However, if there is no egg to be found, the sperm can remain to wait for up to seven days, which means that if ovulation occurs within this time frame, conception is still possible. A mature ovum that has been released can remain viable for up to 24 hours, after which it is no longer fit to facilitate conception. If all of the requirements are met for conception to occur, the ovum and sperm join together. If the egg has not been fertilized within the allotted time frame, the ovaries discontinue producing the two hormones necessary to enable pregnancy, estrogen, and progesterone. While preparing for conception, these hormones assist in thickening the uterus' lining to allow for egg implantation; if the hormones are no longer being produced, both the extra lining and the unfertilized egg are expelled from the body through menstruation.

A zygote is created by the joining of the sperm and the ovum, and the fertilized egg then forms a barrier to prevent other sperm from entering. Beginning with a single cell, the zygote then goes through several rounds of cell division as it goes on its journey of a few days down the fallopian tubes and into the uterus. After four to six days, a blastocyst forms, which is 100 multiple identical cells, and then is all set to be embedded in the uterine wall. Although this is a microscopic ball of cells, some of these cells will not long after making up the embryo and the placenta. After the four-to-six-day period following fertilization has gone by, the embryo begins to fill with fluid, which forms a small cavity. The outer cells begin to build a wall, while the inner cells start to develop into a ball that will eventually become the baby.

It is common to have some spotting as implantation occurs, and the blastocyst is imbedded into the uterine lining. Not long after fertilization does the baby begin to develop all human bodily features, although they are still not discernible with the human eye. The outer part of the blastocyst starts to form the placenta, and the inner parts start forming the embryo. The gender of the child is predetermined much earlier. It is made known to the parents and doctors. A fertilized egg contains 46 chromosomal cells, 23 being from each paren.

The mother's chromosomal cells are abbreviated as XX, while those of the father are abbreviated as XY. The mother can only give X chromosomes, but the father can carry either an X or a Y. The child will be a male (since only males carry the Y chromosome) when the sperm that fertilizes the egg contains a Y chromosome, and if the sperm only contained X chromosomes, then the child will be a female. Within just 24 hours after this happens, the zygote is matured into an embryo. Although the mother may not yet be aware that conception has occurred at this point, the most important thing to consider is your and ultimately your baby's health.

Week 4

In the fourth week following conception, the embryo begins to mature within the uterine lining, and the outer cells link with your bloodstream. At this point, the fetus is less than 3mm long. It has consisted of two layers of cells, and in the fourth week, a third layer is developed. The outer layer, called the ectoderm, forms the baby's skin, hair, eyes, and brain. The middle layer, or mesoderm, forms the kidneys, heart, bones, muscles, and sex organs. The innermost layer, the endoderm, becomes the liver, lungs, and digestive organs. The amniotic sac also begins to form around the embryo and is meant to remain intact until birth.

The amniotic sax protects the child against shock and other hazards. The placenta will eventually function to bring nutrients to and waste from the embryo, but before it is fully developed, the fetus will be sustained by a tiny yolk sac. Once it has matured to a fully operational level, the placenta will enable blood, nutrients, and oxygen to be transferred to the embryo. As all of these drastic changes are taking place inside your womb, other significant changes will occur throughout the rest of your body.

Bodily Changes in the Mother during Week 4

Early on in the pregnancy, you may not notice significant signs except for intermittent tiredness and nausea, which is a result of your body, letting out extra hormones to sustain and develop the baby. Some other symptoms that you may experience could be mood swings, bloating, spotting from implantation, and cramps reminiscent of those that come along with menstruation. It is also possible for slight abdominal pressure to be felt as the embryo is implanted into the uterus. Mammary glands also stimulated to eventually form milk for when your baby is born, which at this point may result in sensitivity or discomfort in the breasts.

CHAPTER 6:

The Seventh Month

This is the third trimester, and things are about to get hot and heavy. This trimester is all about the baby finishing up the development of bones and organs and adding much-needed fat to survive. This growth only begins to crowd Mom's uterus, and those basic daily tasks start to become much more difficult.

This month is important mainly because if your baby were born prematurely, it would have a 96 percent survival rate, which is a wonderful piece of information. Your baby is developing its brain and is finally able to turn its head.

Week 28

Babies born at 28 weeks have an incredible 96 percent survival rate. It's still ideal that they reach full term, but this is just a significant statistic to have at this point. The baby is more than likely moving into a head-down position to get ready for birth. Despite this good news, Mom is having a lot of discomforts these days, with the baby's size and weight causing back pain and pressing on the sciatic nerve.

Baby's Stats

- The baby weighs about 2¼ pounds and is the size of a small eggplant.

- Baby's lungs are maturing.

- Baby is hopefully moving into the head-down position, preparing to be born in a few short months.

- Baby's brain is developing rapidly by growing neurons.

- This is a huge week, as baby's chance of surviving outside the womb if born prematurely, is now 96 percent.

Mom's Stats

- Her internal organs are becoming squished.

- Baby's increased movements mean that Mom is feeling kicks and wiggles more frequently.

- She's likely experiencing frequent backaches and sciatic pain as the baby begins to press on the sciatic nerve.

- She may have shortness of breath as the baby presses up into her lungs.

Week 29

The baby is continuing to grow and gain weight and, at this point, is probably 15 to 16 inches long and around 2½ to 3 pounds. It is beginning to experience REM sleep during its sleeping cycles. Because the baby is growing so quickly, it's starting to get cramped in there, and instead of forceful kicks or punches, Mom will probably start to feel softer blows that are more like jabs and pokes. The other wonderful surprise that might happen around this time is a dampening of the breasts. Mom's body is producing prolactin, which can cause the release of colostrum from the nipples.

Baby's Stats

- Baby has started smiling and is the size of butternut squash.

- Baby is entering episodes of REM sleep and possibly dreaming.

- Baby's bones are mineralizing (hardening).

- The forehead is bulging with a growing brain.

- Baby's current weight is going to double, triple, and the following three months.

Mom's Stats

- Mom's body is producing more prolactin in anticipation of lactation.

- Her belly is growing larger and rounder.

- Her fundal height may be as much as four inches above the naval.

- Her urination has gone from frequent to all the time.

- Her grace in the movement has gone out the window.

- Colostrum may begin to release from her breasts.

Week 30

Your baby is about 16 inches long and close to three pounds at this point. Its brain is rapidly forming, including all of those grooves. Your baby's brain is taking on different tasks now, as well. For the past several weeks, your baby has been covered in fine, silk-like hairs that helped keep it warm. But now the baby's brain can do that, so that hair is slowly disappearing, and it will most likely be gone at birth. Mom's ligaments are relaxing in preparation for the baby's birth, and the size of the baby and uterus is causing all kinds of discomfort.

Baby's Stats

- Baby's brain is getting wrinkled.

- Baby's hands are now fully developed

- Baby is grasping things.

- Fat cells are regulating body temperature, so lanugo is disappearing.

- Baby's bone marrow is now making red blood cells.

Mom's Stats

- Her ligaments are beginning to relax.

- The urge to pee is constant.

- Her breasts have increased in size, and the discomfort continues.

- Mom's lack of sleep causes exhaustion. Essential oils like lavender might be great in an oil diffuser, but you'll need to consult with a holistic expert to make sure you're using something that isn't harmful to the developing baby. Doctors recommend that Mom limit the amount of tea that she's consuming, so that may not be an option.

Week 31

Even though your baby is rapidly approaching birth length and weighs about three pounds, it has another three to five pounds to gain before its debut. Your baby is making a trillion brain connections and already processing information, tracking light, and perceiving signals from all five senses.

Mom is feeling all of those consistent discomforts, and the Braxton Hicks contractions are increasing day by day. Only she can learn and tell the difference between what a Braxton Hicks contraction might be, and then having a baby version, so you've got to stay on your toes and listen to her instincts. Sciatic pain is relatively normal. It happens when the baby is punching, kicking, or resting on the sciatic nerve, causing a shooting pain from the back down through the legs.

Restless legs syndrome is less common (affecting maybe 15 percent of pregnant women), but it is still a real pain in the rear for those who experience it, especially at night when Mom tries to sleep. Acupuncture, yoga, and meditation seem to quell the creeping burning and tingling feeling that overtakes the legs and ruins a good night of sleep.

Baby's Stats

- The baby weighs close to 3½ pounds and is the size of a coconut.

- Baby is now kicking, flipping, hiccupping, and punching the uterus.

- Baby's body fat is increasing.

- Baby can move its head.

Mom's Stats

- Mom's Braxton Hicks contractions increase in frequency and intensity.

- Mom can feel the baby moving, and this can even wake her up at night.

- Mom's discomforts continue.

- Mom may realize when the baby is napping and want to nap at the same time.

CHAPTER 7:

The Eighth Month

You have everything set up to welcome your baby into your home and made it to your final trimester. Your baby will gain about 5 lbs. in weight and will finish their development. While the second trimester might have been a little more comfortable than the first one, the third trimester is often considered the most challenging part of the pregnancy. This is because of the changes in your hormones, your belly's growth, and the labor that will bring you your bundle of joy. While all of this can lead to a change in emotions, the third trimester is a time to celebrate.

During this trimester, you're going to have increased visits with your healthcare provider. You'll go from meeting with them once a month to meeting with them once every two weeks. By the final four weeks of your pregnancy, you'll increase visits to once a week. Make sure you mark the change in your calendar and make your appointments ahead of time so that you can choose the best hours for you.

While you could feel your baby move during the second trimester, in the third trimester, you can see your baby move. Their little kicks flip and flutters can be seen on the outside of your belly as they press against their ever-enclosing space. They'll also manage to maneuver themselves into a head-down position to help with delivery later. If this doesn't happen, your doctor will often give you some exercises that might help the baby move into the right position.

Things to Do During Your Third Trimester

Have a baby shower:

You won't have to plan this yourself, as your friends and family will help, but a baby shower is a great activity to do during your third trimester.

Finish baby's room or sleeping space:

Whether your baby has their own space, or whether they'll be sharing your room, make sure that you finish all preparations. During your third trimester, you may find you tire more easily, so enlist your loved ones.

Finish your birthing plan:

Depending on how your pregnancy is going, you may need to update your birthing plan accordingly.

Plan your route and alternative route to your hospital or birth center:

Knowing how to get to your birthing center or hospital can help when you're rushing off during labor. If you practice the route and some good alternative ways, then you'll automatically know where to go during the high-stress time of labor. Of course, you probably won't be driving yourself, so make sure that your partner or birthing partner also knows (and practices) the route.

Put together a birthing bag, one for you and one for your partner:

Having this ready and waiting by the door once week 36 hits can make things easy as you're rushing through the door to the birthing center or hospital.

Birthing Bag for Mom

Here's a packing checklist you can use to guide your preparation:

- Health insurance and all the forms you need

- Your birthing plans

- A nursing nightgown that opens in the front, and a robe

- Very comfortable shoes and socks

- Toiletries. You can get little travel-sized ones or bring your regular full-sized ones from home. You'll want to bring everything you need for a couple of days

- Snacks and hard candies

- Sanitary pads for heavy flows

- A nursing pillow to support your baby while he or she nurses

- An outfit to go home in. You'll want to choose something you wore in the latter half of the second trimester. Even better if it's something that doesn't press against your abdomen

- Two baby outfits for going home, booties, hats, newborn diapers, and wipes

- Swaddling blankets

Common Symptoms

During your third trimester, you'll likely feel some of the symptoms for your first trimester again. This is because of the change in your hormone levels. Fatigue, mood swings, and reduced energy levels will make a comeback. Here are some other symptoms you're likely to experience.

Increased back pain

Your belly is continuing to grow, and as it does, it's putting more strain on your spine. This back, pain is normal during your pregnancy. It can be remedied by taking pregnancy appropriate pain relievers (talk to your healthcare provider first), taking warm baths, or even getting a prenatal massage.

Your baby might also be pressing against your sciatic nerve, which can cause radiating pain from your back down to your toes on one side. If you're feeling sciatic pain, then talk to your doctor about possible remedies. You can also try sleeping on the other, non-painful side, taking breaks from standing, or getting a prenatal massage.

Hemorrhoids

Unfortunately, the third trimester is when you have an increased risk of hemorrhoids. Hemorrhoids are inflamed veins caused by the changes in your blood volume during the last trimester, or by constipation. They can be very uncomfortable, but there are several remedies you can try. Luckily, once your baby is born, your hemorrhoids will go away very quickly. To help ease the pain, especially if constipation is the cause, increase your intake of fiber, including eating more vegetables and fruit with their skin on. Also, eating more legumes can help. You should also drink a lot of water with fiber to help keep everything moving. You can use some over-the-counter hemorrhoid preparations or witch hazel to help ease the discomfort.

Headaches

With the changes in your blood volume, spine strain, hormones, and blood pressure, you may experience more headaches. You can use regular remedies to combat the headaches, such as a warm compress over your eyes, an ice pack at the base of the neck, and increasing your sleep times. Call your doctor immediately and discuss any other symptoms you're also experiencing if you have a sudden severe headache with changes in your vision.

Sometimes, diet can trigger a headache, so make sure that you keep your blood sugar steady by eating smaller, frequent meals. You should also avoid foods such as chocolate, peanuts, bread, and sour cream, which can trigger headaches. Finally, talk to your doctor about possibly taking Tylenol to help with the pain. Tylenol is generally safe as a pain reliever when you're pregnant, but it's good to first check with your healthcare provider.

Leaking breasts

Your breasts will start to prepare for breastfeeding as your body prepares for delivering your baby, which will lead to some leakage. Even if you're not planning on breastfeeding, your breasts will still leak milk or colostrum. This comes before mature breast milk arrives after your baby is born. The colostrum should be clear, yellowish, or creamy but not bloody. If it is bleeding, talk about it with your healthcare provider. While you can't stop the leakage, you can take some measures, so it doesn't ruin all of your shirts. Insert nursing pads into your bra to soak up the liquid.

Sleeping difficulties

You may notice that sleep becomes harder during your third trimester. Of course, not everyone experiences this, but many women do, as they may feel discomfort from the baby pressing against their bladder, pelvic bone, and the baby's movements. Sleep is still essential, so you should take rest during the day as needed.

Dealing with Emotional Changes

One emotion you'll experience is excitement. You may feel excited about whether the arrival of your baby or no longer being pregnant. You may also feel excited about your upcoming parenthood or wearing your regular clothes again. This can be a great positive emotion during this trimester, and it can help overcome your other emotions. Use your excitement to bolster yourself up when you're feeling low or irritable!

You may also feel some fear about your impending parenthood. The third trimester is when it all becomes real, and you're about to become a parent! This is a fear that may be shared with your partner, so talk about it together. If you're feeling a lot of anxiety about it, consider taking some parenting classes to help you feel more confident about your ability to care for your newborn. You can also find support from other pregnant women, mothers that you currently know, and even from a therapist if you see one. You can also try to write some positive affirmations that can help remind you about your resilience and ability to learn and the love you have for your child. Place them in areas you'll often see, such as on the mirror, fridge, or your phone, so that you can easily see them when you're feeling anxious.

Baby Development

At week 32, your baby has grown to about 16 inches long and weighs over 4 lbs. With this size, you'll feel their movements more as they nudge your uterus to make room. They'll also be growing lovely layers of fat that will insulate and protect them during their infanthood. This is what makes babies so chubby and cute. By week 34, your baby's bones are fully developed, though soft. This helps your baby ease out during delivery, and the bones will harden after your baby is born.

CHAPTER 8

The Ninth Month

At this point in your pregnancy, you have probably gained around 20 pounds or more and probably counting down the weeks to your due date. It is no wonder that you might be feeling exhausted. Fatigue is not uncommon in pregnancy, especially during the 3rd trimester. You might also be feeling some pressure on your organs as the baby grows and moves around. On top of this, your increasing weight might be contributing to your feelings of fatigue as well.

While you cannot get rid of all that extra weight on your body now, you can do several things to help ease your symptoms of fatigue. It can be tempting to give up exercise for the rest of your pregnancy, but it is essential to get moving to help with your fatigue. Exercise is also good for your health. Try to at least walk around the neighborhood every day. Your doctor might recommend that you exercise a little more or a little less frequently, depending on your unique situation.

During your pregnancy, it can be tempting just to eat what you are craving. You might not be thinking as much about the nutritional value that you need to get from your food. Many women are advised to eat six smaller meals a day during their pregnancy. This will help you with feelings of fatigue as well as symptoms of nausea and reflux.

Blurred vision

It may not be spoken of all that often compared to the symptoms of nausea and frequent urination, but believe it or not, blurred vision can happen to you during your pregnancy. This experience can be very confusing on top of all of the other pregnancy symptoms you may be experiencing. Whether or not you decide to get treatment for your inaccurate vision is up to you. Just know that more often than not, this decrease in specific vision is temporary.

While you can get new prescription eyeglasses during your pregnancy, you might want to hold off on getting something more permanent like Lasik surgery until your pregnancy is over. Many times, your eyesight will go back to normal after the pregnancy is finished.

Experiencing blurry vision during your pregnancy is not unusual, but it is still worth mentioning to your doctor. The reason for this is because blurry vision can sometimes be a symptom of another condition related to your pregnancy. Gestational diabetes, preeclampsia, high blood pressure, and pregnancy-induced hypertension are conditions that share blurred vision as a common symptom.

Week 36

At week 36, your baby weighs 6 pounds, is mature, and in a head-down position. The blood and immune system are functional except for the digestion system that will become operational after delivery. For now, the baby relies on your umbilical cord for nutrition, something that will change after birth.

The huge size of the baby does not allow movements, and the Braxton Hicks contractions reduce with time. Pelvic pains may arise as the baby's head pushes your pelvis, and the uterus gets heavier. Pelvic exercises, warm compresses, baths, or massages can help.

Week 37

The baby is heavier than 6.5 pounds, especially if it is a boy; girls tend to be lighter. The baby's head should attain the same circumference as the shoulders, abdomen, and hips.

The downy hair should have disappeared alongside the creamy substance called vernix caseosa. The amniotic fluid continues to reduce as the baby reaches delivery, and the baby's hair rapidly grows to fill the entire head.

The Braxton Hicks contractions may last longer and get uncomfortable; you should also note an increase in mucus discharge from the vagina. The cervical mucus plug helps prepare you for the forthcoming labor. Visit your doctor to check if the cervix has opened enough and its position before you get into labor.

Week 38

The baby continues to shed the Lanugo and vernix into the amniotic fluid, which, when eaten by the baby, forms meconium or the first bowel movement. The fetus is 21 inches long and 7.5 pounds heavy and should now manage a firm grasp at the fingers.

Connections between brain neurons continue to establish.

The baby should have dropped into the pelvis, which makes breathing easier, but still prone to pelvic pains. Most women experience cervix dilation and leaky breast where the breast 'leak' colostrum. It is normal to leak a yellowish liquid from your breasts; therefore, consider placing nursing pads into your bra.

Week 39

The baby continues to produce surfactant- a combination of fat and protein that prevents the lung sacs from sticking to each other after taking the first breaths. Now at full term, the baby is approximately 8-10 pounds and measures 19 to 21 inches. The skin changes from pink to white due to the thick fat layer deposited over the blood vessels. The tear ducts are not open yet, so the baby might not shed tears right at birth.

In some women, the amniotic sac may rupture and release the amniotic fluid; however, this happens only when labor starts. Other signs of labor you might witness include nausea, diarrhea, the loss of mucus plug at the cervix, spurts of energy, and bloody discharge after capillaries rupture at the cervix.

Week 40+

At week 40, the baby does not achieve much growth and is now 6-9 pound heavy and measures 19 and 22 inches. The skull bones are separate, so they can effortlessly compress through the birth canal during labor. For this reason, the baby might have soft spots on the head for the first year. In case you give birth now, the baby's eyes can only focus just an inch away but will recognize you from your voice.

If you reach week 40 while still pregnant, the pregnancy is 'post-term.' Visit your doctor to check for cervix dilation and conduct tests, especially if you hit forty-two weeks without delivering. Watch out for a yellowish fluid that smells like ammonia; this is the amniotic fluid whose rupture means you will give birth within around 24 hours.

Some women can carry the pregnancy beyond 40 weeks; however, past week 40, labor pains can start at any time. See your doctor to check if your pregnancy is still safe and how soft the cervix is.

You may also learn creative methods of speeding up labor and getting into delivery. It is advisable to engage in regular exercises during pregnancy to strengthen the muscles in preparation of labor stress, and to improve endurance during a long labor.

To manage pain during labor, consider doing yoga, walking regularly, changing sitting or sleeping positions, hypnosis, and meditation techniques. You can also listen to music, take a bath, or try out other high-concentration activities. Through good preparation and education, you can choose the best method of managing labor pain.

CHAPTER 9:

Labor and Delivery

L abor and delivery carry its own set of signs and symptoms and things you should look out for. Unlike the three trimesters of your pregnancy, these symptoms are not going to last very long, maybe a few hours to a few days. Some women may experience early labor symptoms for up to a week before labor starts, but these will generally be low in intensity until they get closer to active labor.

Signs of Labor

The following symptoms are signs that labor is preparing to start. These symptoms are generally felt at some point between 37-40 weeks if you carry your pregnancy to term. However, you may experience these symptoms earlier than that if you are going into preterm labor. Better consult your doctor, and they will tell you what to do and when you should come in.

Your Baby "Drops" Into Position

Before labor starts, your baby will "drop" into position. You can tell this has happened when your baby bump is sitting lower down and is more directed towards your pelvis. This is because the baby has officially prepared to enter the birth canal, so they are getting lined up and ready to make an appearance!

Your Cervix Dilates

Probably the most well-known symptom of labor starting in the cervix dilating. Of course, you probably can't tell this is happening, but your doctor will be able to tell you. Your cervix will begin to dilate in the days leading up to your labor slowly. Most women sit around 1-2cm for about a week or two before labor begins. Once labor starts, they will continue opening until they reach 10cm when active labor starts.

Increased Cramping and Lower Back Pain

You may notice more pain in your lower back and more cramping in your abdomen. This occurs due to your muscles preparing to put in all of the work to release your baby. This can also happen because your baby's new position results in new pressures on your lower back and pelvic area. As well, your pelvis will be opening up the last little amount to let your baby come out, so your bones are quite literally stretching open.

Looser Joints

The increased progesterone in your system is still responsible for your joints being loose, though you may notice this even more towards labor. You may experience popping or cracking in your joints a lot more, particularly when you move out of a position you've been sitting in for the same amount of time for a while.

Diarrhea

Many women experience diarrhea leading up to labor. This can be a displeasing opposite of constipation that many women experience in the weeks beforehand. If you experience this, it's just because your muscles are loosening, so are your bowel movements. You have to drink plenty of water and prepare for labor to start.

Your Weight Gain Slows Down, Or You Lose Some Weight

Once your baby is fully cooked, they will pretty much stop putting on weight, because they are getting ready to come out. So, if you notice you've finished putting on pounds or losing a couple, this is why.

You Feel More Fatigued Than Normal

Because of your super-sized belly and all of your hormones, and the frequent need to urinate, it can be hard to get a full night's rest. You may find that you are consistently tired. The best thing you can do is sleep on the side closest to the washroom and keep several pillows on hand to make those few hours of shut-eye restful. As well, rest as much during the day as you can.

You Start Nesting

This is a common symptom of labor that you often see in the media on television shows and movies. Nesting is a symptom many pregnant women experience towards the end of pregnancy to prepare their home for the baby. If you find you suddenly have a burst of energy and all you want to do is clean and get everything ready for the baby to come, it could be because the baby is coming very soon.

Your Vaginal Discharge Changes

Changes in vaginal discharge can include increased or thickened discharge, and a change in color. This is entirely normal.

Your Contractions Become Stronger and More Regular

As your Braxton Hicks contractions change to actual contractions, you may notice they become stronger and more regular in frequency. This is your body preparing to contract the baby out, and unless they are happening minutes apart for a long period, it is completely normal.

Bloody Show/Mucus Plug

As well as your vaginal discharge changes, you may experience your bloody show at some point. This happens as your mucus plug starts to fall out. You may notice a snot-like consistency that is streaked with blood. This is your mucus plug, and you don't need to worry about this unless it's coming out before 37 weeks! Either way, you should tell this to your doctor to be prepared for your impending labor!

Your Water Breaks

Water breaking is one of the most famously known labor symptoms but also happens to be one of the ones that occur the least. Only about 15% of women experience this symptom, and it's usually the last sign that labor is about to start. Once your water breaks, make sure you let your doctor know, especially if it breaks early.

What You Should Expect in the Delivery Room

There are many things to expect in the delivery room, and it varies based on how your pregnancy and labor have gone. If you are carrying a high-risk pregnancy, if you have a scheduled cesarean section, or if something goes wrong and your work becomes an emergency cesarean section, you will have a different experience in the delivery room.

The delivery room is a scary and exciting place, and you may become overwhelmed with emotion while you are there. You are going to be going through a lot, physically and mentally. You are preparing to meet the life you've been creating for the past nine months, and that is a lot to take in! You are likely going to get hooked up to a no-stress-test machine that will make sure your fetal movements are strong and healthy, and to measure your contractions. You are also going to get your cervix checked on a reasonably regular basis, to see how far you are progressing.

A good portion of your stay will be spent relaxing as much as possible so that you have the energy to get through the contractions. You may wish to spend some time in the shower or on a birthing ball to help take some of the pressure and pain of your abdomen. If it gets hard, you may opt for pain medicines, such as laughing gas, or an epidural. If you were GBS positive, you would be hooked up to an IV to get antibiotics every four hours.

Once labor begins, your doctor and a few nurses will come into the room. They will help coach you through pushing and make sure your baby comes out safely. Your doctor may use forceps or a vacuum extractor to help take out your baby if he or she needs a little assistance on the way out. Once your baby is out, your doctor will clamp the umbilical cord and let your partner cut the cord, if you have a partner involved. You will be given a chance to have skin-to-skin contact with your baby and nurse him or her. Sometimes, after your baby has been born, you will also have to push out your placenta, which is not a painful experience for most women and takes minimal effort. The placenta is a tissue, so it will not stretch out your vagina as it exits your body, meaning you will likely not find it painful or painful at all.

The nurses will take the baby for a few minutes to weigh and take some important measurements shortly after your baby is born. You will then be able to shower off and move into a more permanent room where you will remain for the rest of your hospital stay. About twenty-four hours after your baby is born, they will have their vitals taken to ensure that your baby does not have jaundice or anything else. These are called heel-poke tests, and they only take a few minutes to do. Throughout the time you are there, your nurses will come in to check on you and your baby to ensure that you are both getting along well, and provide you with any support or assistance you may need along the way.

CHAPTER 10:

Expecting Multiples

News of upcoming twins, triplets, and other multiples indeed a thrilling and great surprise for any couple. Disbelief, pride, and panic are just a few of the feelings you might experience on the road to parenting multiples. Not to mention the physical ramifications of having more than one baby on board. Your pregnancy may mean more frequent visits to the doctor and a higher-maintenance prenatal routine, but the joys of being a multiples' mom make it all worthwhile.

Splitting Eggs and Sharing Sacs

Multiples are either monozygotic (formed from a single egg and sperm) or dizygotic (created from two separate eggs and sperm). Monozygotic multiples, more commonly known as identical, can be further classified by sharing their shared space and material resources.

Your Body in Multiples' Pregnancy

You are living more extensive than you ever imagined. With all those arms and legs flailing about, you feel like you're housing a team of tiny Olympic hopefuls. Although it may not feel like it when your crowd is going wild, and your back is killing you, a multiples' pregnancy is a unique gift. That your body can accommodate and nurture not just one, but two, three, or possibly more human beings is nothing short of miraculous.

Moms-to-be of multiples experience the same pregnancy symptoms as women with only one fetus, but these can be more intense and occur earlier in the pregnancy. In particular, excessive nausea and vomiting are often an early sign that your unborn child has company. However, many women with singleton pregnancies can experience severe morning sickness as well. More significant markers of multiples' pregnancies would include the presence of more than one fetal heart tone during a prenatal examination and measuring too large for your suspected gestational age after week 24.

High levels of alpha-fetoprotein (AFP) on an AFP, triple screen, or quad screen blood test can indicate that you have some stowaways. Doctor's Visits

If you've been diagnosed with a multiples pregnancy, you'll be visiting your doctor more frequently. Although your appointment schedule will depend on your specific medical history and the risk factors involved in your pregnancy, you might be visiting twice monthly in early pregnancy (as opposed to just a monthly visit for the first trimester with singleton pregnancies). Then you will shift to weekly visits early in the third trimester.

Diagnosis

While some symptoms and screening tests point to a multiples' pregnancy, a definitive diagnosis is usually made by ultrasound. During the ultrasound procedure, the technician will try to determine whether or not the fetuses share a single amniotic sac since this can put them at higher risk for some complications.

Do You Need a Perinatologist?

A perinatologist is an ob-gyn who specializes in high-risk pregnancies — is a good choice for many women expecting multiples. If your medical history is complicated or if you are expecting triplets or more, the expertise of a perinatologist can be quite valuable. When choosing a perinatologist, it should also be someone with whom you feel comfortable and able to communicate. There may be a specialist in the practice your original doctor or midwife belongs to, making the transition easier.

Problems in Multiples' Pregnancies

Multiple pregnancies have a shorter gestation time than singleton pregnancies, simply because mom hasn't enough room and resources to house the brood for forty weeks. On average, twin pregnancies are usually delivered at week 38, triplets at week 35, and quadruplets at week 34. The most significant risk by far in a multiples' pregnancy is preterm labor and premature birth. Gestational diabetes and preeclampsia are also risking.

Problems Mom May Face

If your body is nourishing two or more children, you need to treat it with a little extra TLC. Take an additional 600 calories daily of healthy foods (beyond average pre-pregnancy calorie intake), and drink plenty of water. The latter is particularly important since dehydration can trigger preterm contractions.

Moms-to-be of multiples are at higher risk for developing anemia and should speak to their provider about iron supplementation to ensure that their needs are covered. Increasing your intake of iron-rich foods is an excellent way to ward off anemia. Try rotating iron-fortified foods such as baked beans, blackstrap molasses, wheat germ, raisins, beef, and leafy green veggies (like spinach, kale, and broccoli) into your diet. The cervix has heavy work to do in a multiples' pregnancy. Having twins puts you at an increased risk of preterm labor. Some physicians have recommended serial screening of the cervical length using transvaginal ultrasound to try to detect early cases of preterm labor.

A screening of the cervical length at around week 20 appears to be predictive of who will deliver preterm. Some reinforcements may be required in women with a short cervix (approximately 25 mm or less at week 24). If cervical shortening is suspected, a transvaginal ultrasound in which the Doppler wand is inserted into the vagina rather than moved across the belly is used to assess the cervical length and monitor the cervix's progress. Cerclage, a procedure involving suturing (or stitching) the cervix closed to avoid preterm dilation, is not routinely indicated for multiples' pregnancy but is sometimes performed for preterm cervical shortening and dilation.

Problems Babies May Face

Up to 70 percent of monoamniotic twins and higher-order multiples experience umbilical cord knotting, twisting, or entanglement. In severe cases, kinks or tangles in the cord can cut off blood supply to both fetuses. Ultrasound can determine the presence or absence of a dividing membrane between multiples. If a multiples' monoamniotic pregnancy is detected, it will be followed closely with routine ultrasounds to check for umbilical cord complications. Regular non-stress testing (NST) may also be employed to evaluate fetal health.

Delivering Multiples

Nothing is routine in a multiples' pregnancy, and the surprises will likely keep coming through labor and delivery as well. Communicate with your health care provider and a neonatologist (a physician who specializes in newborn and preemie care) about the possible scenarios you and your children face at birth will make you better equipped to make informed decisions.

Cesarean Versus Vaginal Delivery

About half of all twins are born via cesarean section, and the number goes up considerably for triplets or more. Because of the risk of umbilical cord entanglement, multiples that share an amniotic sac are usually delivered by C-section at or before week 34.

Whether other multiples are delivered vaginally or not will depend on how they are positioned in the womb. If the first baby is breech (feet or buttocks first), your provider will probably prefer a C-section. If at least the first baby is vertex (head down), vaginal delivery may be performed. Women who feel strongly about having a vaginal delivery of their multiples should speak with their provider early on in the pregnancy.

A quick ultrasound in the labor and delivery room will reveal your babies' positions. In some cases, when the first baby is born but the second is breech, the external cephalic version may be attempted to turn a stubborn twin. The fetal heart rate in the second twin will be monitored during the procedure.

CHAPTER 11:

CHAPTER 11:

Postpartum: The First Week

B eing prepared for what's to come in labor, birth, and life after baby can be empowering. It's also important to be ready for the unexpected. Go with the flow when your birth plan or postpartum plans can't always be achieved in the way you envisioned.

Here are some specific things that you can do to improve outcomes of labor, birthing, and postpartum recovery:

- Take a birthing class.

- Decide how detailed (or not detailed) you want to be with your birth plan.

- Have a support system in place. Consider if a doula would be a good fit for you.

- Understand your options for labor and birthing positions and breathing and pushing patterns.

- Prep your perineum and pelvic floor for this big event.

Recovering from childbirth is unlike anything else—your hormones are surging, the body is healing, and on top of that, you have a tiny human to take care of.

Perineal Massage

Typically, 35 weeks of pregnancy is a good time to start focusing on relaxing and lengthening the pelvic floor muscles and getting the vaginal opening used to pressure and stretch. There is some evidence to suggest that performing perineal massages for a few minutes a week can be beneficial to decrease tearing during childbirth.

Typical recommendations are performing the massage or stretching for one to five minutes, anywhere from three times daily to at least once a week.

Steps to Perform A Perineal Massage:

- Get in a comfortable position. Imagine your vaginal opening as a clock: noon is up towards the clitoris and 6:00 down towards the anus.

- With a clean finger (and potentially using some lubricant or oil), you or your partner can insert one finger about an inch into the vagina at the 6:00 position. Gently stretch downwards for up to a minute. You may want to start with 10 to 15 seconds and build up a tolerance.

- You can also gently make your way from the 6:00 position towards the 3:00 and 9:00 as if making a U for a few minutes.

- You could enter two fingers and stretch outward and down at the same time.

It should be noted that working on any older scar tissue in the perineum or cesarean scars is also a great idea. You can do this before getting pregnant again, while pregnant, or postpartum.

It is recommended that you use the compression support of your choice during the day of your first week and take it off at night to give your body a break. In the second week, start to decrease the use of it when you're up and moving more (roughly 50 percent of the day). By the third and fourth weeks, wean off the compression and feel more of your core strength beginning to activate. Wear 25 percent of the time during periods of more activity.

From day one postpartum and for the next few weeks, it's essential to rest and let your body heal. Consider staying off your feet for the first few weeks. Ask for help if this recommendation feels far-fetched. Spend time in bed or on the couch healing. Aim for rest and ask for help to achieve this in the early days. Perform gentle breathing exercises. When you do need to exert yourself (getting up from sitting, rolling over in bed, lifting baby), exhale to decrease pressure on the pelvic floor, and make it easier to move. Set tiny goals to increase your activity tolerance slowly. This portion of exploring your new life with a baby should be taken seriously to allow your body to heal. Be intentional with your mind and body.

Continue to listen to your body, postpartum for the signs and symptoms. There may be days you feel ready and restored to get back out there, and there may be days and weeks where your body screams rest. Your mindset and choices in the movement should be intentional, with an emphasis on breathing and pelvic floor strategies. Do what you can to find a balance and continue with self-care.

Postpartum: The First 6 Weeks

When you reach the time of the six-week checkup, speak up if things don't feel right and if you have questions about how to function in this new body and life of yours. Six weeks is not a magic number and ask for help if you have concerns. And maybe you feel fine at six weeks, but symptoms arise later at six months. Speak up then. It's not too late.

You should have your 6-week checkup with your doctor or midwife following delivery. They check how the tissue is repairing and healing, making sure that there are no signs of infection and that your uterus is healing properly. It's more than just getting clearance for sex and exercise. While it's important to know whether your body is ready for these activities, it's also important to have other symptoms evaluated.

You should have your 6-week checkup with your doctor or midwife following delivery. They check how the tissue is repairing and healing, making sure that there are no signs of infection and that your uterus is healing correctly. It's more than just getting clearance for sex and exercise. While it's important to know whether your body is ready for these activities, it's also essential to have other symptoms evaluated.

Lab	Evaluation
Complete Blood Count (CBC)	Evaluates white blood cells, red blood cells, and screen for anemia.
Ferritin	Evaluates iron stores.
Comprehensive Metabolic Panel (CMP)	Evaluates liver, kidney, and gallbladder function.
Thyroid Panel (TSH, Total T3, Total T4, Free T3, Free T4, Reverse T3)	Evaluates thyroid function and health.
Thyroid Antibodies (Anti-TPO, Anti-Thyroglobulin)	Screens for autoimmune postpartum thyroiditis.
Vitamin D	Determine vitamin D status and evaluate if supplementation is warranted.
B12 and Methylmalonic Acid	Evaluates vitamin B12 status.
Folate	Evaluates folate status.
Homocysteine	An indirect marker of inflammation that also gives insight into B vitamin utilization.
MTHFR Gene	Evaluate if there are underlying genetic issues that may affect mental health, energy use and detox pathways.
HgA1C	Marker of blood sugar over a 3-month period. Important if you had gestational diabetes.
CRP and ESR	Measurement of inflammation
Salivary Cortisol	Determines function and health of adrenal glands.

Natural Relief for After Birth Pains

After birth, pains are normal, and they can be pretty extreme for some women. They are the result of your uterus contracting back to its original size, a process known as involution.

These contractions begin about 12 hours following delivery and may be as mild as your menstrual cramps or as intense as labor contractions. Each time you nurse in the early days following birth, you will also feel these contractions. This is because the baby's nursing stimulates the release of oxytocin, often called the "cuddle hormone," which causes contractions and helped return your uterus to its original size, among other things. Another benefit of breastfeeding!

In addition to returning your uterus to its original size, these contractions prevent excess bleeding, which is why it is important to avoid aspirin. Aspirin thins the blood and can lead to increased bleeding.

If you feel like you need to take something for these contractions, try to avoid acetaminophen or ibuprofen as these have side effects that can impact your health, such as leading to intestinal irritation. Instead, keep the following remedies near you when you breastfeed to alleviate pain:

Homeopathic Mag Phots 6C.

Take 3-5 pellets every 15 minutes for pain. You may find it helpful to take a dose just before you begin nursing.

Hot Water Bottle.

Apply heat up to 20 minutes to the small abdomen. Wrap the outside of the hot water bottle with a towel and avoid making contact with the baby.

Cramp Bark (Viburnum opulus) Tincture.

Take two droppers full just before you, nurse. It reduces pain without inhibiting the uterus from shrinking.

Motherwort (Leonurus cardiac) Tincture

Take two droppers full up to 4 times daily. Motherwort is a uterine tonic that eases anxiety, irritability, and supports a healthy heart.

Uterine Massage.

Every time before you stand up for the first 3-6 weeks postpartum, massage your uterus. Make your hand into a fist and knead the lower belly. This is a technique that may help decrease the amount of bleeding and helps the uterus heal.

Natural Remedies to Heal Urinary Tract Infections

Urgency, frequency, or pain with urination may be signs of a urinary tract infection (UTI). It's better to contact your doctor if you experience these symptoms, especially if you have a fever, nausea, backache, or blood in your urine. If caught early, you may not require an antibiotic. However, if there is any risk of the infection affecting your kidneys, you want to act quickly and meet with your doctor. A medicine will be necessary to resolve the disease and protect your kidneys.

Prevention:

- Wear white cotton underwear changed daily
- Use only mild, natural detergents on clothing
- Use non-deodorized, preferably organic, sanitary pads
- Wipe front to back after a bowel movement
- Avoid bubble baths
- Shower after swimming
- Avoid tight pants
- Eat Lacto-fermented foods three times weekly

Diet:

Avoid sugar, alcohol, caffeine, aspartame, and dried fruits until symptoms resolve.

Increase Water Intake: Drink a glass of filtered water every 20 minutes for 2 hours, then every hour for 24 hours, except during sleep.

Vitamin C: 1,000 mg 4-5 times daily for two days. It can cause loose stools, so decrease the dose if this occurs. After two days, reduce dose to 500 mg 4-5 times daily for five days.

Cranberry Juice: Drink 4 ounces of unsweetened cranberry juice four times daily for one week.

Cranberry D-Mannose: 2 capsules twice daily for one week.

CHAPTER 12:

If You Get Sick

Pregnancy is never easy even when you do all the right things and take care of your body and mind, you will still experience days when you feel ill, your emotions seem uncontrollable, or your back is aching terribly. Although these issues may make your pregnancy less comfortable, they can be partially remedied. These are all typical aspects of a healthy pregnancy and mean that your body is doing the right things in preparation for your new baby.

Sometimes more severe medical issues arise during pregnancy that, if left untreated, can put the health of you or your baby in jeopardy. Thankfully, modern medicine means that we have many tests and methods to diagnose such events and treat them accordingly. One of the reasons it is so important to attend all of your scheduled medical appointments during pregnancy is to detect any abnormalities and address them early. Although any pregnant woman may experience an unexpected health concern during her pregnancy, the chances significantly increase if you are in a high-risk pregnancy.

What Is A High-Risk Pregnancy?

A doctor refers to a high-risk pregnancy when there are potential complications that could affect the mother, the baby, or both. If your doctor deems your pregnancy to be high risk, it will likely mean that you will need to have additional tests and appointments, and may need to meet with a specialist, depending on the specific situation. You can rest assured that your doctor and other medical professionals will manage your job to ensure the best possible outcome for you and your baby.

There are several reasons for which a pregnancy may be deemed high-risk. The most common of these is maternal age. Generally, women under the age of 17 or over the age of 35 when their baby is born are more likely to experience complications during pregnancy than those aged between 18 and 34. Women who are very young during pregnancy are more likely to have their baby early, which often means that the baby is born underweight. If you fall pregnant during your teenage years, make sure you pay special attention to your diet, as keeping your baby well-nourished is essential to ensure healthy growth and development. Focus on leafy green vegetables, whole grains such as brown rice and quinoa, and lean protein sources like grilled chicken.

As maternal age increases over the age of 35, so too does the risk of several complicating factors occur during your pregnancy. The risk of miscarriage is higher for older women, and the chance of a baby being born with a genetic defect increases significantly after the age of 38. For decades, scientists have known that advanced maternal age increases the risk of having a baby with a genetic abnormality, but the reasons for this link are still being established. When a baby girl is born, she already has every egg–or oocyte–her body will ever produce. It is theorized that oocytes become vulnerable to changes in and degrade the DNA they contain over the time they spend in the ovaries. In other words, eggs in the ovaries for 40 years are more likely to have unstable DNA that could lead to a genetic defect compared to those that have only existed for half that time.

The most common example of this is Down syndrome, a condition characterized by intellectual impairment, developmental delays, and physical abnormalities. Each cell in our body is supposed to have two copies of every chromosome, but Down syndrome occurs when a baby is born with three copies of one particular chromosome, chromosome 21. Down syndrome cases range in severity of the symptoms, and those affected by this condition experience varying degrees of quality of life, and usually a shortened lifespan. Thanks to advances in genetic technology, genetic screenings during pregnancy are now available for Down syndrome and tests for some other genetic defects.

What Is Genetic Screening and How Does It Work?

Despite the increased risk of a complicated pregnancy, more women than ever choose to have a baby later in life. This is partly due to societal changes and the fact that many women prefer to establish a career before starting a family. However, it's also partly due to the great medical advances that have been made in recent years, reducing the risk of a complicated pregnancy, and allowing women to wait until they are ready to start a family safely. One such advance has been genetic screening, the ability to take a sample of a baby's DNA before it is born to test for many different genetic conditions. Genetic testing, also referred to as chorionic villus sampling (CVS) when performed on a fetus, usually occurs between weeks 10 and 12 of pregnancy. This procedure involves removing a small piece of the placenta, which is then sent away for genetic analysis.

Importantly, genetic testing isn't just for your baby. If a specific hereditary condition runs in your family, such as cystic fibrosis, there's a chance you could carry this disease in your genes even though you don't have the disease. This means that (although the chance is usually small), you could pass this onto your baby, who may be affected by the condition, particularly if your partner is also carrying the gene. Genetic testing gives you the ability to have your, and your partner's DNA analyzed to assess your baby's chances or risks of passing on a hereditary condition.

Genetic testing can be very beneficial if you are of advanced maternal age. It can provide you with the peace of mind that your baby doesn't have any of several common conditions or can prepare you for what may lay ahead. However, it's an entirely personal choice and does come with a small risk to the baby since it is an invasive procedure.

Understanding Gestational Diabetes and Preeclampsia

Gestational diabetes and preeclampsia are the two most common complications during pregnancy. Gestational diabetes is a type of diabetes that first develops during pregnancy and is typically detected during the middle of the pregnancy. Doctors usually test for gestational diabetes between weeks 24 and 28. It is essential to test for it because if the condition is diagnosed, steps must be taken to ensure the safety of both mother and baby. A pregnant woman diagnosed with gestational diabetes cannot adequately regulate her blood sugar levels. If the mother has high blood sugar, this can also cause the baby's blood sugar to be high. This can result in complications, such as the baby growing too large and the potential requirement of a cesarean section birth.

Preeclampsia is distinguished by high blood pressure, protein in the urine, and persistent swelling in fingers and toes. It can cause preterm labor and result in complications during labor, such as a seizure or stroke. Although this condition is severe, with proper diagnosis and monitoring, there's no reason why a pregnant woman with preeclampsia can't have a normal birth and a healthy baby.

Managing Complications

For some expecting mothers, gestational diabetes and the resulting complications occur during pregnancy for seemingly no reason. However, you can make several easy lifestyle changes to help reduce your risk of gestational diabetes, unregulated blood sugar, high blood pressure, and preeclampsia.

Pay careful attention to your diet to reduce your risk of developing gestational diabetes. Eat healthy, nutritious foods such as fresh fruits and leafy green vegetables), whole grains such as brown rice and quinoa, and lean protein sources grilled chicken or fish. Avoid very fatty foods such as bacon and sugary foods such as cakes and desserts. Eating well will help to keep your weight gain in check, which will reduce your risk of developing gestational diabetes.

If you do improve this condition, you can help to regulate your blood sugar levels by following a meal plan designed for someone who has diabetes. Your doctor or a nutritionist will be able to provide you with an idea of what to eat if you develop gestational diabetes, which will likely focus on the foods mentioned above. If you develop gestational diabetes, it's essential to avoid foods that are high in sugar like soda, fruit juice, and cakes or pastries, as these will cause a very high spike in your blood sugar levels.

Exercise can also play an important role during your pregnancy. Regular exercise before and after you fall pregnant can lower your risk of developing gestational diabetes. Yoga helps balance food intake, keeps blood sugar levels stable, and ensures that your weight stays healthy. If possible, aim for 30 minutes of moderate-intensity physical activity at least five days a week, or as much as you can manage. Remember to focus on non-weight bearing activities such as brisk walks, swimming, yoga, and cycling.

Make sure you monitor the condition regularly if you develop gestational diabetes. Measure your blood sugar levels often, as instructed by your doctor, and record the results. You will need to take them at different times of the day and before and after you have eaten. If necessary, your doctor may prescribe insulin for you to take. Make sure you take this as instructed, as it will help regulate your blood sugar levels to keep your baby healthy.

For most women, gestational diabetes resolves soon after giving birth. However, a small subset of women develops type 2 diabetes as a result of their gestational diabetes. If you have had gestational diabetes, make sure you get tested for diabetes 6 to 12 weeks after giving birth, and then every two years. Even if your gestational diabetes does go away, you are at an increased risk of developing type 2 diabetes later in life, so continuing to eat healthily, exercise regularly, and be tested frequently is essential.

CHAPTER 13:

Pregnancy Loss

The probability about 15-20% of pregnant women can face a miscarriage in their pregnancies. Here are the following causes:

Age of the Mother.

It can affect pregnancy. Miscarriages are quite rare in these ages, usually below 30 years old. A woman is at her great health for carrying a child but as the woman gets older, the risk of miscarriage gets higher, because of her age.

Placental Problems.

The placenta is where the mother is linked to her child through the blood supply. When there is a problem with the blood supply in the placenta, the pregnancy could be threatened by abortion

Chromosome Problems.

Chromosomal problems usually cause miscarriages that happen during the first trimester of pregnancy.

Chromosomes are the human "building blocks," and human beings have 23 chromosomal pairs; each chromosome is derived from either parent. When there is an insufficient pairing that occurs during the union of the sperm and egg, a miscarriage could become an issue.

Infection.

Late miscarriages often result in the health of the mother. Usually, when a late miscarriage occurs, it is due to an infection in the womb that causes the water to break or the neck of the uterus to open prematurely.

Blighted Ovum.

At times, there will be noted successful implantation in the ovum, but no baby is formed. This case is often related to chromosome problems. In this case, the woman will appear pregnant, but during pregnancy, all the symptoms will stop, and vaginal bleeding will occur.

Medications.

The use of certain medications can also increase the risk of miscarriages. Take note of the following drugs and their purpose:

- methotrexate – for rheumatoid arthritis

- non-steroidal anti-inflammatory drugs – for pain and inflammation

- misoprostol – for rheumatoid arthritis

- retinoids – for acne and eczema

Increased Caffeine.

Caffeine is a common chemical that functions as a stimulant. It is found in food, drinks, and medications and is often related to cases of miscarriage. Pregnant women are advised to either stay away from caffeine or limit their intake to just 200 milligrams per day. Take note that one mug of tea contains 75mlligrams of caffeine, and one cup of coffee contains 100milligrams of caffeine.

Womb Structure.

The structure and development of the womb can also affect pregnancy. Some second-trimester miscarriages are related to any abnormalities in the womb which includes problems such as:

- fibroids. Non-cancerous growths that can grow outside or inside the uterus

- cervical incompetence. This refers to a weakened cervix or weakened muscles of the cervix (also known as the neck of the womb) which is usually related to injury from surgery or early opening of the cervix

- The abnormal shape of a womb. This can be caused by the bones of the pelvis being misaligned. The bones will then push on the uterus and cause it to become abnormally shaped. The abnormal shape can cause the baby to be mispositioned inside the womb, such as transverse position, breech position, or the most common frank breech. Chiropractic care is highly effective at aligning the pelvis, therefore returning the uterus's shape to its normal form. All pregnant women should be under Chiropractic care for this reason and many others.

Polycystic Ovary Syndrome (PCOS).

This is a leading cause of infertility in women, and when a woman can get pregnant, the condition can threaten the child. While its direct role in miscarriages is quite unclear, there is some connection, so it is worth noting.

- Progesterone Deficiency.

- It is believed that women who are found to have low levels of progesterone are at risk of suffering a miscarriage. Supplements can be taken to remedy this progesterone problem but note that there is no real guarantee that supplementation will prevent the miscarriage.

- The Health of The Mother.

- As the mother carries the baby throughout pregnancy, the mother's health is crucial and is often instrumental to the success of the pregnancy. The mother's doctor should note the following to prevent problems related to this, so that they may be addressed before the pregnancy can progress:

- Hormone problems. If there are inefficiencies in the production and secretions of certain hormones, it may affect the pregnancy

- Diabetes. The body's ability to manage blood sugar can also affect pregnancy. More so, diabetes is noted to be related to the maintenance of the health of various body organs such as kidneys, blood vessels, eyes, and nerves.

- Thyroid disease. The body utilizes energy from food to carry out its functions. The thyroid glands help in the storage and utilization of said energy, so it is vital. A mother with thyroid disease is health compromised, and her pregnancy is put at risk because of this.

- Autoimmune disorders. When a pregnant woman is suffering from an autoimmune disease such as lupus, it means that her body is not working well to protect her from it. This means that the body cannot defend itself from infection, so the baby's life is highly at risk.

- Infection. The presence of disease during pregnancy can compromise the mother's health and the child. Examples of these infections are rubella, cytomegalovirus, Chlamydia, syphilis, HIV, bacterial vaginosis, gonorrhea, and malaria.

Note that these are causes that could be pinpointed for this misfortune.

But it is essential to know that miscarriages can never be related to the mother's emotional status during pregnancy, stress, depression, an instance of shock or fright, exercise, lifting or straining, work and sex.

It is a misconception that these things can lead to a miscarriage.

CHAPTER 14:

Coping with Your Miscarriage

Miscarriage can be one of the darkest experiences in pregnancy. Coping with a miscarriage in a constructive and healthy approach is to remember you are not to blame, and you are not being punished for anything. Be kind to yourself and during your period of grief.

The following are ways to help you through these dark days of grief and help you understand that there is hope after a loss. Not everything works for everyone as everyone copes differently; remember there is no right way or wrong way to grieve the loss of a pregnancy. Find places, people, and resources to help you on your grief journey.

General Coping Mechanisms

Your grieving process is your own.

You don't have to do it on anyone's timeline but your own. If you can, tell people what is happening. This doesn't mean you need to lay your heart out on the table every time someone asks how you're doing it. This just means if you feel brave enough to be honest about your emotional state, you should be. Some people might find it hard to listen because no one likes to see someone care about in such pain, but this will also give them an insight into where you're at in your grief journey. They can't extend compassion if they don't know how you're feeling. If you're acting like everything is okay, they will act like everything is okay. They will be taking their cues from you.

Gather the women in your life around you.

Women you care about love and can find comfort in. They don't need just to be family; they can be aunts, grandmothers, and close friends. You need women you can trust. Women you can cry with. Women will just understand this pain from a different perspective than a man might. Healing will start when you find yourself in a group that can comprehend your loss on an intense and intimate level.

Do not let your grief and loss create a divide between you and your partner.

This is truly a time where you and your partner need to be a team as you both process your grief. Though you may go through your grief journeys differently, you can support one another in a way no one else can. You both have experienced a loss, and you help each other cope. Do not rush the process even if those around you start saying things such as "get over it" or "you just need to snap out of it and move on." You will move on when the moment is right for you and not anyone else. This is about what works for your process. Don't rush the process; trust the process. Your feelings are your own, and you need to own them and understand whatever you're feeling at whatever time is normal. If you need it, seek professional help to get through this.

Don't forget to take care of yourself.

While taking care of others during their grieving process might help you cope, you must be careful not to become a way for you to forget about yourself. Do not let this happen, as ignoring your grief will only lead to being swallowed up by it. It's incredibly important to remember to eat, sleep, shower, and leave the house even when you don't want to. These everyday tasks will seem pointless and hollow, but it is essential to be persistent as this routine will help you in the long run.

Sex with your partner will be different at first.

Expect sex to be a little strange at first. Some couples do try to conceive very soon after a miscarriage, and while this is fine, you should consult your doctor first. Also, remember if you feel the need to take a break from trying to conceive, that is perfectly alright. But sex will be unavoidable that at some point. You might find that the act of lovemaking is intimidating because it is what led to the pregnancy, which can lead to such pain and heartbreak. It is alright if your attitude towards sex changes. It may even, just for a little while, change radically. The key here is the fact that you should be honest with your partner when this happens. Make it clear you aren't rejecting them but that your feelings about the act of sex have changed.

Understand as well that just unexpected as a miscarriage is, the emotions and grieving process that occur in the days and weeks and even months that follow are just as unexpected. There may be a day when your loss is not the first thing you think of when you wake up in the morning or the last thing you think about when you go to sleep at night. The best thing to do is just to go with the emotions. Acknowledge them and allow them to happen. Shutting them out might lead to a much bigger emotional collapse later on in your grief journey. There will be days of triumphs and days where you are completely unsure if you can get out of bed. Your emotions will ebb and flow, but eventually, they will even out, and you'll come out the other side of this emotional rollercoaster and look back on how far you've come. As you persevere, you will learn to face the world calmly and hopefully again.

Active Coping Mechanism

The grieving process isn't the same for everyone. While some may deal with their miscarriage by talking it out and gathering loved ones around them, others might cope in more physical or active ways as they process their miscarriage.

Try doing something creative.

Some research suggests that creative pursuits such as painting or drawing or playing a musical instrument help soothe the brain's emotional centers. Whether it's writing in a journal or dancing to a favorite song, these creative outlets can help with the grieving process.

If you know how to sew or perhaps know someone who does create a memorial quilt might also help you through your grieving process. Whether you choose to display it afterward or just have it as a keepsake, building the quilt will allow you something creative and constructive to do while processing your emotions as you pick fabrics and shapes.

Journaling.

Some women who have experienced a miscarriage find journaling to be a great help, especially when they are not yet ready to talk about it, or they just want to sort out their feelings. It can be a great outlet during the grieving process.

Get fresh air.

When a person is grieving a miscarriage leaving the house can often seem like a daunting task as it allows the person to avoid any possible grief triggers. But stepping outside, even into the backyard for a moment or two, can help clear a person's thoughts and re-energize the body.

Associate with a hobby to keep your mind occupied.

In the early stages or after a miscarriage, a person often feels like all they think about is the loss of their pregnancy, but in the later stages, some might be looking for ways to not think about it. It is an excellent opportunity to look into a new hobby or activity. This will allow you to focus on something other than your loss and will enable you to meet new people who know nothing about your miscarriage and won't always be on your guard about whether they'll ask about your grieving process.

CHAPTER 15:

Cesarean Delivery

Many times, we go into the pregnancy, assuming we will have a vaginal birth. This is generally seen as a healthier option to help your baby come into the world and thrive. But at some point, you may find your baby needs to be delivered through c-section. Sometimes this is planned ahead of time, and you and your doctor can schedule the procedure ahead of times. Other times you may already be in labor at the hospital when your doctor decides to do the c-section.

C-sections are relatively common in the United States right now. About 32 percent of babies are currently being delivered by c-section, which means you have a one in three chance of having to go this route for one way or another. While any surgery is something that should be taken seriously, you can feel better knowing this is a standard procedure done to keep you and your baby safe. There are different reasons why the c-section is scheduled for you and your baby. In some cases, the doctor may discuss doing this procedure with you ahead of the due date and then will schedule it with you. A few factors to help your doctor determine whether a c-section is necessary ahead of time or not includes:

Certain medical conditions:

If you are dealing with conditions that could make a vaginal delivery stressful on the body and birth difficult, then the c-section may be a safer choice. Some of the conditions which could be considered include kidney disease, high blood pressure, diabetes, and heart disease.

Infections:

If the mother is HIV-positive or has an infection of genital herpes, which is active, then the c-section could be scheduled. This ensures the baby doesn't get those two diseases when they are delivered.

The health of the baby:

A congenital condition or an illness could make an already tricky journey out even worse for the baby.

A large baby:

Sometimes, the baby could suffer from macrosomia. This is when the baby is too large to make it through the birth canal safely. This can happen in cases where you gained more weight than is recommended during pregnancy.

Your weight:

Being obese can significantly increase your chances of needing a c-section, usually because of some of the other risk factors which can show up when you are obese, like gestational diabetes. This can sometimes be because obese women tend to have longer labors, which can increase your risk of being on the operating table.

Your age:

While being of an older age doesn't guarantee a c-section will happen, the odds of having one can increase with your age.

Breech position: If the baby ends up being butt first or feet first and can't turn them around, your doctor may discuss whether the c-section is necessary.

Problems with a placenta:

If the placenta ends up partly or entirely blocking up the cervical opening, or it separates from the uterine wall, it may be safer for the baby and you to undergo a c-section.

Other complications:

There could be some other complications which would make a c-section more likely. If you develop preeclampsia, high blood pressure due to pregnancy, or eclampsia, a condition that can cause seizures, and the treatment doesn't seem to work; it may be best to go with a c-section.

A previous c-section in the past is sometimes possible to do a VBAC or vaginal birth after c-section but having a c-section in the past will increase your chances of having another one.

If your doctor is talking about doing a c-section and wants to get one scheduled, make sure to ask a lot of questions. Check if there are any other options, and at least have a full understanding of why your doctor is interested in it.

In most cases, when a c-section occurs because something comes up during the labor. The woman and her doctor had planned on a vaginal delivery, but the need for this procedure didn't show up until the woman was well into the labor process. The reasons for this could include:

Labor doesn't start:

If you can't get the labor to start moving, and you aren't dilating even though you are having contractions, after 24 hours, then your doctor may decide to go for a surgery.

Labor stalls:

You may get started on the early stages of labor, and then stall there. Sometimes oxytocin or another option can start the contractions up again, but if it isn't helping, then it may be time for a c-section.

Exhaustion or fetal distress:

If you are in labor for a long time and the doctor determines you are becoming exhausted, or the fetal monitor shows signs of distress in the baby, then it may be time for this procedure.

A prolapsed umbilical cord:

If the umbilical cord starts to slip into the birth canal and the baby isn't there first, it can become compressed as the baby comes out. This can cut off the oxygen supply to the baby.

Elective C-Sections

Since these kinds of deliveries can be safe and will also help prevent the pain of labor, some women prefer to do this procedure over doing a vaginal delivery, and they may ask for this in advance. However, these numbers are dropping due to the 2013 policy statement from the American Congress of Obstetricians and Gynecologists. This group recommended the doctor and the mother always plan for a vaginal delivery unless there is some medical reason for a c-section.

Many doctors and other medical professionals have been pushing to lower how high the c-section rates are in the United States. This can help keep the baby safe, remove the need for a surgery that could be unnecessary for many mothers, and promote a quicker recovery time. Even though a c-section is a very safe and routine procedure, it is still major surgery, and there are some risks to you and the baby. When you and your doctor plan on a vaginal delivery for the birth, unless a medical reason shows up, you are giving yourself and your baby the best option.

What to Expect During The C-Section

Most hospitals are going to try and keep the c-section procedure as safe and comfortable as possible. If possible, they will keep the mother awake, allow her partner to be in the room, and they provide the mother with a chance to meet and cuddle with her baby right after the delivery, as long as there is no reason medically not to. Since you aren't going to be busy with the pain or the pushing, you can relax and marvel at the birth a bit more.

A c-section will begin with some routine IV and some anesthesia, usually either a spinal block or an epidural. This helps the lower half of the body to stay numb, but you will still be awake. Then there will be some prep work done with the stomach being shaved if needed and then washed with an antiseptic solution. The operating room staff can then insert a catheter into your bladder and place some sterile drapes over the stomach. Your partner or another individual in the room will be given sterile garb and then allowed to sit near you and hold your hand.

The staff will place a screen between your head and stomach to ensure the area stays clean and ensure you won't watch the cutting process.

In some situations where an emergency c-section is needed, there may not be time to numb you, and the general anesthesia will knock you out for the procedure. This is a rare case, and since the procedure only takes a few minutes, you won't be out for long. When you do wake up, you may feel a bit sick to your stomach, disoriented, and dizzy.

Once you are asleep or numb, the doctor will get to work and place a small incision in the lower part of the abdomen. It could feel a bit like the skin is being unzipped, right above the hairline. With some neat suturing, the scar isn't going to be too noticeable, and it can fade more over time. Then the doctor is going to make another incision to the lower part of your uterus. For both of these incisions, there two main options a doctor can go with.

The two options include:

A low transverse incision:

This will be a cut going across the lower part of your uterus. This is often done in most c-sections because the muscle found at the bottom of the uterus is seen as thinner, which means less bleeding. This muscle is less likely to have any tears or problems if you have a vaginal delivery later on.

Vertical cut:

This is the incision going down the middle of the uterus. This is the one that is used if the baby nestles itself low into the uterus or ends up in another unusual position.

The amniotic fluid will be suctioned out, after which the baby will be pulled into the world. There is the possibility of feeling a bit of tugging at this point. Since the mucus found in the baby's respiratory tract didn't get all squeezed out during the birthing canal's journey, there may need to be extra suctioning to get it out and hear the first cry.

The surgeon will remove the placenta after the umbilical cord is cut and do a quick check of all the reproductive organs to make sure they are still working well. The doctor will then stitch you up with some absorbable stitches in the uterus, the kind they won't have to go through later, and take out, and then there will either be some surgical staples or stitches in the abdominal incision. This part is going to take about 30 minutes or longer to finish.

At this time, you may also get a few other things. The doctor could give you some antibiotics to help reduce your risk of infection. You may receive some oxytocin in your IV to control the bleeding and properly help the uterus contract. Your pulse rate of breathing, blood pressure, and the amount of bleeding you have will be checked regularly.

When all of this is done, you will get some time to spend with the baby. Some women can nurse on the operating table, but you can at least do it in the recovery room. You will have plenty of time to bond with the baby, and breastfeeding will happen if you don't sweat it too much.

Recovering from A C-Section

Often, the recovery process of a c-section is going to take longer than with a vaginal delivery. While you may be ready to start caring for your newborn, this procedure's emotional and physical recovery will take longer. You will need to spend about three to four days at the hospital, and then it can take up to six weeks at home to get back to normal. Slow and steady is the best thing after this procedure. You are already going to be taking care of the baby, don't try to strain yourself too much. Remember that c-section is major surgery, and you need to give your body the time it needs to do well and heal.

CHAPTER 16:

Postpartum Depression

A s a new mother, you only hear about the joys of motherhood. You hear about what it feels like to meet your baby for the first time, the bond that you have. What happens when your experience is not like this at all? Maybe you deliver your baby, only to realize that you are very depressed, not connected to anyone. If this happens to you, know that this is a normal condition experienced by many mothers worldwide. This is postpartum depression, and it is a common condition for new moms to develop. No matter how much you have been looking forward to having your baby, the postpartum depression can still rise to the surface before you realize what is happening.

There is not only a single reason why you might develop the condition, but there are a few prominent factors. Hormones can have something to do with it. After you give birth, your estrogen levels and progesterone levels experience a big drop. When you have been living with elevated levels for nearly a year, your body gets used to this. As these hormones drop, your thyroid function can also drop. This is what leaves you feeling depressed and sluggish. Changes in your blood pressure, immune system, and metabolism can all trigger your experience with postpartum depression, as well.

What is the Difference Between PPD and Baby Blues?

A common condition that mothers develop after pregnancy is the baby blues. This differs from postpartum depression (PPD) because it is not as serious. Immediately after childbirth, it is common for the new mother to experience at least a bit of baby blues. This has something to do with the sudden change in hormones in your body, but it can also be combined with the stress experienced during delivery. After giving birth, everything seems to be moving very quickly for you and your new baby, causing you to feel overwhelmed and fatigued. Don't worry because this is bound to change very soon. Once you get used to your routine, you will usually be able to beat the baby blues.

When you have the baby blues, you might feel extra emotional in the days to follow your delivery. This can mean more tearful moments and more emotional fragility. Know that this is perfectly normal. You will notice a peak in these symptoms after one week postpartum, but then you can expect them to taper off by the time that you enter the second week. This is a good indication that what you are experiencing is the baby blues. It should not last much longer than this. If it does, you might need to consult your doctor to determine if you are suffering from PPD.

You can think of the baby blues as mild depression, whereas PPD is more severe depression. When you have mild depression, mood swings are still common. One moment, you might be happy to be spending time with your baby and your family, and then that feeling will subside and become replaced with stress or anxiety. This is new for you, so don't forget to give yourself plenty of time to breathe. Needing a break does not make you a bad or weak mom. Ensure that your partner plays an equal role to prevent either one of you from feeling burnt out. Your partner can help you a lot during times when you feel that you have the baby blues. By picking up the slack, you won't be left feeling quite so overwhelmed.

What Are Recognizable Symptoms?

PPD is something that should not go ignored. Because it is a more intense form of depression than the baby blues, you might need to consult your doctor for a solution. When you have PPD, you will experience a wide range of symptoms. Pay attention to the severity of each symptom that you feel and see if you can relate to these. Some of the most common symptoms are the following:

Withdrawing:

After giving birth, you probably imagined that you would feel closer to your new family than ever. Every moment leading up to the delivery showed you that you would be spending plenty of time enjoying your baby and bonding with your partner over the new arrival. You might be experiencing symptoms of withdrawal if things do not go as planned.

No matter who you are withdrawing from, your baby or partner, this is a sign that PPD might be occurring. If you feel that you cannot bond with your baby or are no longer close with your partner, know that this feeling will pass with the proper treatment.

Anxiety:

When you have anxiety that is out of control, it will impact you mentally and physically. You might not be able to eat or sleep, which makes it much more difficult to take care of your baby. To provide them with nourishment, you need to be taking the best care of yourself. Your mind will run wild with the what-ifs, torturing you into thinking that you aren't doing a good job.

Even when your baby appears fine, like eating or sleeping, you might be second-guessing yourself and wondering why you are doing everything wrong. This type of anxiety can place a lot of unrealistic expectations on you, preventing you from enjoying this time that you have with your newborn.

Guilt:

You might experience feeling washed over by guilt after you give birth to your baby. You might feel guilty over how you delivered your baby or how much you can give them now that they are born. These thoughts will keep cycling through your mind, making you preoccupied.

When you have intense guilt, this can make even the most enjoyable moments stressful because you are constantly worrying. It is easy to move past the guilt and focus on the positive sides, but PPD makes this part difficult. This might prove to be a feeling that you cannot shake.

Worthlessness:

It can be very hard to experience worthlessness when you have a new baby to care for. They depend on you for everything, from nourishment to shelter. On the inside, all you might be able to feel is that your life no longer matters. On some days, you might even wish that you could just disappear altogether.

This reaction tends to come with the fact that you are already very stressed out. Raising a baby is not easy, but this does not mean that you are worthless because you are trying your best. No mother has all of the answers, so you should not expect yourself to have them.

Suicidal Thoughts:

One of the most serious symptoms of PPD is suicidal thoughts. Just because you have PPD does not automatically mean that you will develop these thoughts, but you must look out for them. Becoming preoccupied with death, or wanting to die, is very dangerous and should be reported to a medical professional. If you are experiencing this, do not delay telling someone and getting help.

The sooner you open up to someone you trust, the sooner you will feel relief from your PPD symptoms. Motherhood is not all stress and worry. You can enjoy your life in your new role. Lean on your partner for extra support when necessary. Look at your baby, remembering that you brought them into this world. You completed a huge task already, and you are wonderful for doing so.

Best Coping Strategies

There are ways to cope with your PPD, no matter how severe it gets. When you prioritize taking care of your baby, this automatically means that you must take care of yourself. What you can provide for your baby is a direct extension of what you can provide for yourself. While this time is going to be difficult for you, know that this is not what it will feel like forever.

Create a Secure Attachment:

Known as an attachment, this is the emotional bonding process that occurs between you and your baby. To create a secure attachment, you have to pay attention to your baby. When they are feeling discomfort, try to soothe them right away. After they start crying, offer them solutions, whether they are cuddles or feeding.

Your baby is going to feel secure when they know that you are always there for them. It is a way to build trust that your baby will understand, even as an infant. This is how you will set yourself up for a great relationship with your baby as they grow older. It will also show you that you have plenty of purpose and reason to be there, as PPD can often trick you into feeling otherwise.

Lean on Others for Help:

You don't have to keep your feelings to yourself. If you don't want to admit exactly how you feel to your partner, consider opening up to another mother. You would be surprised at how many other mothers have also dealt with PPD and successfully overcame it.

Even if you don't want to go very in-depth, it helps to have emotional support. Anyone who appears supportive in your life right now should be someone you are spending time with. Don't forget to prioritize these relationships in your life.

Take Care of Yourself:

After giving birth, you shouldn't have to jump back into doing all of the housework. Let your partner take care of this, as you need to take care of your body. While the first thing you might want to do is make the house as perfect as possible, put yourself first. Make sure that you are fully healed before you get back into any kind of physical activity.

When you do start feeling better in a few weeks, you can get back into low-impact exercise. This involves walking and doing gentle at-home workouts. The endorphin rush will help you combat your PPD. By exercising, you will also be getting better sleep at night. This is essential for any new parent and practices some mindfulness meditation to clear your head.

Make Time for Your Partner:

Your partner has now been filled with ways to take care of your infant—this is natural, but you don't want to let your little one takes over every opportunity you get with your partner. Keep your relationship strong during this time. You will both need mutual support.

When your baby is asleep, check-in with your partner, see how they are doing and what they are feeling. You both know the experience best, as you are raising the same child. Don't forget to engage in intimate moments together. Even if you don't feel like having sex yet, cuddling, kissing, and hugging is a great way to re-enter the intimacy.

Seek Professional Help:

If you feel that you cannot handle your PPD on your own, commend yourself by taking the big step. Your doctor will be able to help you in a few ways. One of which is attending individual therapy or marriage counseling. Talking to a professional can be enough to ease your mind. When you can get the worrisome things off your chest, you are making more room for happiness.

Antidepressants or hormone therapy might also be recommended to you. No matter which is recommended, your doctor will be keeping a close eye on you to make sure that you are reacting well to the medication and that you are safe.

CHAPTER 17:

How to Deal with the Morning Sickness

N ausea can be one of the main reasons you might be afraid of going through the ups and downs of pregnancy. Morning sickness is a complaint of more than half of all pregnant women and finds it annoying.

It remains at its peak around the sixth week, and you can blame it all upon the four hormones estrogen, progesterone, HCG, and cholecystokinin.

It might also be the outcome of a lowered blood sugar level culminating due to the placenta's call for energy. As suggested by researchers, morning sickness is a good sign, and it brings with it the good news that your pregnancy is at a lower risk.

Nausea is just a name that adds insult to the injury and nothing else. Here are the tips to get along with it.

Breakfast in Bed Can Heal

Nausea will be the first thing to deal with as soon as you wake up with a low blood sugar level and an empty stomach, worsening the case. Getting up and moving all-around your house won't do you any help. Eat your breakfast in the bed and bite them slowly. You are recommended to stick to dry products like cereals and toast, which will surely not be your first choice but will help boost your blood sugar level and help the body gain calories quickly.

Eat Less but Eat Frequently

Having your food frequently and taking them in smaller portions can help you get along with this feeling. The acids produced by the stomach have nothing to work upon except for the stomach lining, in case your stomach is empty. This is the main reason why you feel nausea. Frequently eating will benefit you by stabilizing your level of blood sugar. Have foods like bananas that are rich in potassium at breakfast to comfort you against nausea. Bland foods like salty crackers are preferable. Help your body by sticking to foods like nuts and cereals rich in protein to maintain the blood glucose level, especially at night.

Keep Your Body Hydrated

Staying hydrated is crucial for you and your baby. On the one hand, it feels like a challenge to consume about 8 cups of water in a day as your stomach will not be ready to keep anything down, and on the other, dehydration can aggravate this feeling. Try sipping six glasses a day and crunching on potato chips that trigger your thirst. You can even add honey or apple cider vinegar to make your drinking water palatable. Fruit juice can also be a good choice. Avoid caffeine-rich, sugary drinks like coffee and soda.

Breathe in Fresh Smell

You become super sensitive to smell when you are pregnant. Estrogen is again to be accused of as it is responsible for the sense of smell. It makes you have the radar nose, which means you may now feel like throwing away your favorite meal because of its smell. Avoid letting in heavy odors like perfumes, tobacco, and vehicle exhaust and escape as soon as you get them. Try sniffing at the satisfying smell of lemon or rosemary whenever required.

Get Yourself a Good Sleep

Nausea is directly related to fatigue. It increases when you are stressed out. You are required to provide yourself the rest it needs as it is working extra to grow your baby. Get an undisturbed sleep at night to combat nausea. You can even take short naps in the daytime but try to avoid sleeping straight after the meal as it increases nausea. Keep your work aside if it is complicating your nausea. Rest whenever you are tired and see how it works wonder for your physical and mental well-being.

Keep Yourself Fit

Feeling sick? Go for a walk around your block. It is the best idea to be thought of when you are pregnant as it helps to get your blood moving. A short walk for about twenty minutes, preferably after breakfast, can help you with digestion and is also known to release endorphins, which helps counteract the feeling of nausea. Keep yourself busy by reading books, solving puzzles, and watching televisions. This will serve by protecting your mind against negative thoughts.

Also, being vocal about your emotions and sharing thoughts with your loved ones can boost you up and help by alleviating morning sickness.

Vitamins Are Vital

Try not to let the morning sickness go out of your hand and consult your doctor if you face a tough time. If you have a problem with anti-nausea medicines, try substituting them with vitamin B6 only after being supervised by the doctor. Vitamin B6 helps to diminish the feeling of nausea. Doctors mainly recommend folic acid for the first trimester.

Get Yourself an Aromatherapy

Ginger has always been praised for its ability to suppress your queasy. It helps by settling your stomach. You can add a slice of ginger to the water or tea or sip a cup of ginger ale. Snacks that are made using ginger such as ginger cookies or gingerbread can go a long way in helping fight nausea. Exposure to the scent of peppermint has also been noted to decrease the level of nausea.

Start Wearing Comfy Clothes

Your body needs to be caressed in comfortable clothes. Avoid wearing tight clothes as it will only worsen the matter. Most pregnant women easily accept clothes that are of loose-fitting. It is found in studies that moms who experience nausea had fewer symptoms when asked to wear loose and comfortable clothes. You can avoid sweating and getting hot flashes by wearing loose cloth and letting the cool breeze in.

CHAPTER 18:

Welcoming Your Little One

After all of the preparation you've done changing your priorities, getting mentally and physically ready for baby, and buying baby items, now comes the time to welcome your new baby into your home. Ensure that you bring the car seat to the hospital when you go in to deliver and pack a bag for yourself and the baby.

Prepare change of clothes for yourself and a robe and remember a camera for pictures. You'll want to capture those first moments of life. For the baby, pack an outfit for him or her to go home in. Also, bring a baby blanket. You won't need to bring diapers because the hospital will supply you with them during your stay.

Your House

Before you go into labor, set up your baby's bedroom. Put the crib together. Set up the dresser and put away any clothes you have for him or her. If you have a changing table, set that up too. Also, clean the house so that it's freshly sanitized. That way, you won't be frantically cleaning when you bring your new baby home, and he or she won't get sick from any leftover germs. Another good idea is having meals prepared for the first couple of weeks.

Even freeze some things that you can thaw so that the food will last for two or three weeks. That is if you don't have anyone to help you by bringing over anything. It will just make the transition welcoming your little one into your home that much easier.

Utilizing Your Support System

Let certain people on your list of people call to know when you go into the hospital to deliver. That way, they can plan to come and help you when you bring your baby home. Like I said earlier on, don't invite everybody over the first few weeks. You don't want too many people in your house when you're adjusting to having your baby home.

Just one or two people who will be helping out. Helping you prepare meals or clean. Maybe watching the baby while you get some rest to recover from delivery.

Enjoy Your Baby

After preparing and welcoming the baby into your home, you adjust to a new way of life. Don't forget to enjoy every stage. Time goes by, and your little one will grow so quickly. Enjoy changing diapers and late nights up, putting him or her back to sleep. Soon, the baby will be in the toddler stage, and you'll be dealing with toilet or potty training. Enjoy it all. You only get one chance at them being small so, please make the most of it.

Being a Parent

Congratulations on becoming a new parent. It is one of the most amazing but difficult experiences in life.

Relationships as A New Parent

When you become a parent you often put a tension on relationships with your partner, friends, or family. But there are ways you can work through tough times and stay close to your loved ones. You can get very emotional and upset quite easily in the first few days after birth, generally known as the 'baby blues,' it is normal and happens to most new moms.

Let your family help you out as much as possible, especially if you are lucky enough to have your mother help you and reassure you.

Sex and Contraception for New Parents

Don't feel rushed into sex! Babies and small children can get in the way of your sex life. You're often tired and stressed, and there aren't many opportunities for intimacy. You and your partner may be happy with the situation. Still, if your sex life becomes a problem, a lot of tender loving care and patience, and some changes will be needed, intimacy is important and doesn't always need to be sexual. You and your partner will need to use contraception if you're not planning to have another pregnancy.

Keeping Healthy as A New Parent

Every new parent will tell you that it is exhausting, and you may have no time to eat properly, exercise or energy to cook. But being active can help you relax and can also help your body recover after childbirth and make you feel better and more energetic. And eating well doesn't need to take lots of time or effort.

Coping with Stress as A New Parent

Small children require a lot from you, and their very lives depend on you. Dealing with their demands and everything else that's going on around you can be stressful, sometimes joining a club for new mums helps, you get to find out you're not the only one struggling. Ask for help as this is where family and extended family usually love to help out with a newborn, the baby is their family.

Number one priority, though, is to look after yourself; you can't look after your baby if you are not on top form too. Proper nutrition is a great place to start whatever stage of life you are at, making sure you eat well, exercise, and take relevant supplements for the breastfeeding stage. Take a general multivitamin for yourself once the little one is weaned and children's vitamins for your little one.

CHAPTER 19:

Baby Sleep Problems

Newborns and Small Babies

At this age, you must accept a degree of disrupted sleep. It will pass, but my best advice is to give yourself a break. As I've said earlier, take all the help you are offered, don't give yourself a hard time about a messy house or a takeaway dinner, and know that it will soon be over, and everyone will be sleeping better. Just rest, enjoy your newborn and recover from the birth and pregnancy. It's honestly not for long. There are a few sleep issues you may come up against that you may want to address for safety reasons or because they will make your life easier and aren't difficult to fix.

Not being able to sleep on their back

At this age, it's recommended that babies are always put to bed on their backs, as any other position increases the risk of SIDS. One solution is to swaddle babies firmly in a blanket to help them feel secure and stop them from flailing. Another is to rock them gently to sleep, then move them into their bassinet or cot once they are deeply asleep. If you are consistent, she will eventually get used to sleeping on her back.

Not knowing the difference between night and day

Babies have no sense of night or day and frequently wake throughout the night. We've looked at ways you can start to give them a sense of night and day, which will help over time. These include going outside and getting some natural light in the daytime and keeping nighttime waking as dark and quiet as possible, so she gets the message that darkness is for sleeping.

Hunger

If you are breastfeeding, be sure to keep in touch with a lactation consultant to ensure that your baby is getting a good feed, as a hungry baby will find it hard to sleep. You may need to hold your baby or feed for a long time to get them off. Always get as much help as you need, and you can look forward to better sleep once the feeding routine is established.

With bottle-fed babies, again, ensure that the baby is getting enough food, checking the instructions for mixing the formula up carefully. A warm bath, followed by a feed, should provide a good sleep.

Two to Three-Month-Old Babies

Sleep regression

Around this age, your baby should be sleeping better. However, you may also notice a sleep regression. This often accompanies a growth spurt or development leap and is characterized by an alert, active baby who shows no signs of wanting to sleep. Setting your nighttime routine – bath, story, bed – so that your baby gets the message that nights are for sleeping, not playing. It will soon pass, but if you exhaust, see if you can get some extra rest or naps in the meantime.

Feeding through the night is another habit you can fall in to, especially with breastfed babies. Your baby feeds little and often, leaving you exhausted. If you keep your baby in your room with you, you may be able to manage night feeds without fully waking up. But if you would like to stretch out the time between feeds, so you get more sleep, try and give your baby a good feed last thing at night. Perhaps express a bottle of milk so your partner can take over one feed (although this may be more hassle than it's worth, and some breastfed babies will simply refuse a bottle and hold out for the breast. Creating set times for bottles or breastfeeds in the daytime and trying to stick to them may also guide your baby towards a more regular sleeping and feeding pattern.

Teething pain

Some babies may seem unsettled when they have a tooth coming through, with red cheeks and drooling. Extra cuddles, a teething ring, and a warm bath will all help to settle him. Teething will generally pass quickly, but if your baby seems to be particularly unhappy, visiting your family doctor is worth a try. They may recommend some baby painkillers, which will help with sleep, too. Teething can also be used as a catch-all term for any unsettled behavior. Sometimes, it's worth looking a little deeper to discover if there are any other solutions to unsettled behavior.

Four to Five-Month-Old Babies

Overstimulation

Around this age, your baby may drop a nap and start sleeping less in the daytime. This may lead to her being overtired at night and harder to settle. It's important to realize that an overtired baby may 'fire up' and become much more active, loud, and energetic than sleepy. This can be a sign of overstimulation, so if your baby seems overtired, try starting the bedtime routine a little earlier with all its associated sleep cues so they can catch up on sleep.

Sometimes, with an overtired baby, it takes longer for them to wind down, which can create a vicious circle of another late night followed by another unsettled day. It may help to 'break the cycle' with a busy afternoon that includes some play and outside time, followed by a good feed, a long bath, and an early bedtime. No matter how alert your baby seems, keep in mind ideal sleep quantities for each age bracket and aim to get them – very tired children won't learn and thrive as well as well-rested ones.

Six months

Still waking up wanting a feed

Although we don't remember it in the morning, we all wake up during the night a couple of times and fall back to sleep again almost immediately with no memory of the event. Babies need to learn to fall back to sleep, preferably on their own without requiring too much help from their caregivers, past the age of about six months.

If you've been feeding your baby to sleep, you might now consider moving this feed to thirty minutes before bedtime and following it with a board book story and some lullabies in bed. You can expect some fussing at this change of routine, but if you are consistent, she will drift off without the bottle or breast if she is tired. Hopefully, this will make night-waking easier – if she learns that she can get back to sleep without a feed, just your voice and perhaps a gentle stroke should be enough to settle her again.

Of course, if you don't mind feeding through the night, don't feel you have to do this. But if you are exhausted during the day, it might be a good idea to introduce some gentle sleep training around six months to make day-to-day life easier.

Early waking

Some babies wake early, raring to go. You can try adjusting naps and bedtimes or put a black-out blind over the window to try and push her wake up time back a little. Another option is to bring her into your bed and hope that she drifts back to sleep.

Ultimately, though, early mornings are part and parcel of having a young baby, so getting to bed earlier yourself so you can handle the early start may be the best solution.

CHAPTER 20:

Tips for First-Time Mothers-To-Be

First Trimester

Find the right doctor for you.

Even if you made a few visits to your ob-gyn or have been going to the same one for the last five years doesn't mean that you are the right one for you and your baby. Explore your options, visit different doctors, and choose the informative one and the one you are most comfortable with.

Do not read pregnancy forums on the Internet that scare you.

Some pregnancy materials are scary to read, and then there are also Internet forums where experienced mothers share their horrific experiences or believe that there is something with what you are feeling. Stay away from it if you are feeling anxious. If you feel like something is wrong, make a quick call to your doctor and refrain from searching the condition on the Internet.

Purchase a nightlight for your bathroom.

You will find yourself peeing a lot, especially during the first trimester and the third trimester. Install a nightlight to make it easier for you to navigate your bathroom without slipping or stepping on anything that might make you fall.

Don't go overboard shopping for maternity clothes.

Yes, you will still want to look good while pregnant, but it's more important to save your money than to spend it on maternity clothes that you probably won't wear a lot anyway. Your body will continually change throughout your pregnancy if you feel your clothes becoming snug, buy 1 or 2 maternity pants or dresses, and wear the hell out of them. When you reach the second and third trimester, your belly will still enlarge, requiring you to purchase different maternity clothes set.

Find a support system.

Pregnancy can be hard, stressful, and overwhelming, so seek the solace of people who make you feel better and have your best interests at heart.

Second Trimester

Take a trip.

During your second trimester, you will start feeling slightly better, and the frequency of getting morning sickness will be reduced. This is the perfect time to take a trip with your partner or with your friends. It is a great way to relax.

Cross off significant items on your to-do list.

Frequently review your to-do list during your second trimester and do your best to cross them off. This will also be the best time to finish the tasks you should have done in your first trimester. So, prepare your baby room, finish household projects, complete your baby items, and come up with a budget.

Take childbirth classes.

Childbirth classes are high, and they can provide you with the information that you'll need to ensure a healthy delivery.

Sleep a lot.

Sleep early, and if you are feeling a bit tired during the day, then sleep.

Check your maternity clothes.

You are probably more prominent now compared to your first trimester. Before you go on another shopping trip, ask your friends or family if you can borrow some clothes. It is essential to save money when you are pregnant, so try to be resourceful as much as possible.

Third Trimester

Ask for help.

Everything will become a bit harder once you reach the third trimester. You will have some trouble putting on or removing your shoes, and you will have difficulty standing up, find it hard to get in the car, etc. But you mustn't hesitate to ask for help. It is better to kindly ask others than to risk harming you and your baby.

Relish the last few months that your baby is in your belly.

Savor the bonding moments you and your baby have and the different sensations you feel when you move inside you.

Place a waterproof pad underneath your bed sheet.

Now that you are due any minute, the body might go out of control with things that you cannot prevent. You might accidentally pee your bed, your water might break, or your boobs might leak. Having a waterproof pad underneath your bed sheet will make it easier for you and your partner to clean, and you can even use it again under your baby's sheets.

Stock up on essentials.

Prepare big meals that you can quickly heat when you are hungry, stock up on your baby's necessities like diapers, milk, and clothes, have a lot of underwear ready, buy lots and lots of baby wipes, stock up on fruits and vegetables, etc.

Conclusion

You are now a mom, and the journey has not been easy, but the smile that your baby puts on your face wipes away all the agony you went through. Becoming a mother is a dream come true to most women. Welcoming a baby into your life strengthens the bond you have with your partner.

Carrying your baby for nine months and successfully delivering it calls for a celebration. You are a first-time mother. There are plenty of new things that you have learned throughout your pregnancy. Some of the lessons learned will be handy for the rest of your life. In the childbirth classes, for example, after giving birth, some of the things you were taught will help raise your baby as recommended.

Now that your baby is next to you and you are feeding or spending time with him or her, the last thing that you want to remember is the uncomfortable feelings that you had to go through during the first few weeks of your pregnancy—lower back pain, vaginal bleeding, mood swings, bloating, and headaches. The worst thing about these symptoms is that you never knew what was going on. Accordingly, it must have been difficult for you to decide whether or not to call a doctor since the experience was your first time.

Usually, after learning that you are pregnant, you don't expect any more spotting. However, you may have later come to realize that the spotting was because your follicle was rupturing. The point here is that the constant worry about whether your baby is okay has finally been rewarded with a special gift. Due to your naivety, the chances are that you wanted to schedule an ultrasound during the first three weeks. Nevertheless, an ultrasound scan will not help you see anything in your belly. This is because it was too early to scan.

One important thing that you should always bear in mind is that your pregnancy will depend heavily on how well you take care of yourself. This entails having a weekly checklist to remind yourself of the most important changes happening to you and your baby. Every week, you should be aware of what is going on inside your belly. During the second and third trimester, your awareness will guarantee that you know when things are okay and when to call your doctor.

Undeniably, the first trimester will be unbearable. Usually, this is the point where most women get easily irritated due to their mood swings. Since your partner might also be new to the experience, you must talk to them about your bodily changes. Keeping them updated will keep them to your side, and they will understand your sudden mood changes. Concerning sex during the first trimester, your partner must comprehend why you keep pushing them away. It is a common pregnancy symptom for women to have a low sex drive during the first three months. Therefore, this should not be a reason to fuss.

Another huge concern that could worry you during your pregnancy is whether it is safe to exercise. The reality is that exercising is of great benefit for you and your baby. There is no reason to laze around at home with the perception that you will harm your baby if you work out. You should consider engaging in light exercises such as walking, cycling, and swimming, etc. When approaching the late stages of your pregnancy, always ensure that you are not straining yourself. It is prudent to do some light exercises as they make a huge difference in your health.

Of course, you will also be worried about gaining weight when carrying your baby. Well, this is part of the process. Don't fall for the myths that a tiny baby will be easier to deliver. Stick to a balanced diet and provide your baby with the nutrients it needs for optimal growth. You will have plenty of time after delivery to tone your body. Your baby's health depends on you, so don't let them down.

It is also vital to remind you about the importance of a birth plan. You will be dealing with concerning your pregnancy, and you should consider writing a birth plan. This plan details some of the most important things that should occur when your baby is due. For instance, this document will reveal some of the preferences that you have in mind about whether you will have a C-section. Additionally, a birth plan will detail essential items that should be packed in your hospital bag. Such minor details are often overlooked, and it could lead to a huge inconvenience if your baby decides to show up unannounced.

Your baby's movements during the second and third trimester will hint a lot about your baby's well-being. This is perhaps the best way of interacting with your baby and knowing if they are okay. Your baby will be kicking, rolling, and fluttering inside you. What happens when you suddenly notice that they are no movements? Does this mean that your baby is sleeping or that they are tired? You must notify your doctor or midwife about any irregularities in your baby's movements.

You should watch out for labor symptoms during the latter stages of your pregnancy. Often, these symptoms can be confused with the common symptoms that you might have been experiencing. When you start noticing that nesting instincts have kicked in, this could be a good sign that you are almost due. Make good use of these signs to start preparing early to welcome your baby into this world.

Your doctor, midwife, or your general practitioner should be your best friend for 40 weeks. This means that they are there to provide you with any form of assistance you need. Therefore, you should always consult them and express your concerns without any worry. Have fun raising your baby.

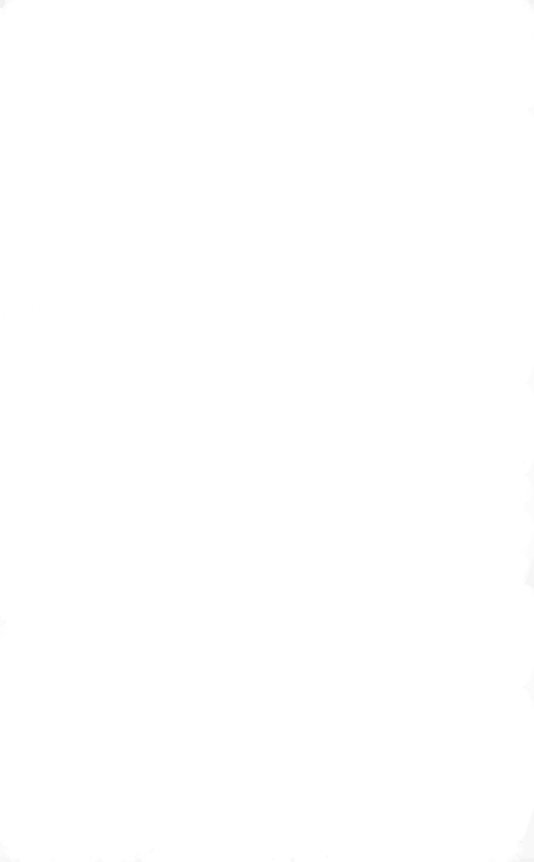

CPSIA information can be obtained
at www.ICGtesting.com
Printed in the USA
BVHW091944300121
599169BV00002B/406